Gold Medal Nutrition

FOURTH EDITION

Glenn Cardwell, APD
Nutrition Impact Pty Ltd

HUMAN
KINETICS

Library of Congress Cataloging-in-Publication Data

Cardwell, Glenn, 1956-
   Gold medal nutrition / Glenn Cardwell. -- 4th ed.
     p. cm.
   Includes bibliographical references and index.
   ISBN 0-7360-6069-3 (soft cover)
   1. Athletes--Nutrition.   I. Title.
 TX361.A8C35 2006
 613.2024'796--dc22   200503022

ISBN-10: 0-7360-6069-3
ISBN-13: 978-0-7360-6069-1

Unless otherwise noted, data for tables with nutrition information came from the following sources:

Food labels

Food company Web sites

Food Standards Australia and New Zealand. 1997. Nutritional values of Australian foods. Canberra: Australian Government Publishing Service.

Food Standards Agency. 2002. *McCance and Widdowson's the composition of foods.* 6th summary ed. Cambridge: Royal Society of Chemistry.

Pennington, J.A.T., and J.S. Douglass. 2005. *Bowes and Church's food values of portions commonly used.* 18th ed. Baltimore: Lippincott Williams and Wilkins.

The Web addresses cited in this text were current as of January 2006, unless otherwise noted.

Acquisitions Editor: Michael S. Bahrke, PhD, **Developmental Editor:** Christine M. Drews; **Assistant Editor:** Maureen Eckstein; **Copyeditor:** Patsy Fortney; **Proofreader:** Anne Rogers; **Indexer:** Gerry Lynn Messner; **Permission Manager:** Carly Breeding; **Graphic Designer:** Nancy Rasmus; **Graphic Artist:** Yvonne Griffith; **Photo Manager:** Sarah Ritz; **Cover Designer:** Keith Blomberg; **Photographer (cover):** Marco Garcia/Getty Images; **Photographer (interior):** Sarah Ritz, unless otherwise noted; **Art Manager:** Kelly Hendren; **Illustrator:** Malcolm McGill (cartoons); all other art by Craig Newsom, unless otherwise noted; **Printer:** Versa Press

10 9 8 7 6 5 4 3 2 1

Human Kinetics
Web site: www.HumanKinetics.com

United States: Human Kinetics
P.O. Box 5076
Champaign, IL 61825-5076
800-747-4457
e-mail: humank@hkusa.com

Canada: Human Kinetics
475 Devonshire Road Unit 100
Windsor, ON N8Y 2L5
800-465-7301 (in Canada only)
e-mail: orders@hkcanada.com

Europe: Human Kinetics
107 Bradford Road
Stanningley
Leeds LS28 6AT, United Kingdom
+44 (0) 113 255 5665
e-mail: hk@hkeurope.com

Australia: Human Kinetics
57A Price Avenue
Lower Mitcham, South Australia 5062
08 8277 1555
e-mail: liaw@hkaustralia.com

New Zealand: Human Kinetics
Division of Sports Distributors NZ Ltd.
P.O. Box 300 226 Albany
North Shore City
Auckland
0064 9 448 1207
e-mail: info@humankinetics.co.nz

This edition is for members of my favourite team—
Toni, Kitri, Zane and Leah

contents

foreword

I can clearly remember the first time I met Glenn, nearly 16 years ago. I quickly found that we had lots in common (including the love of chocolate and Australian football) and I had lots to learn from him (how to be a good communicator and educator). He stands out as one of my favourite sports dietitians—and not just because he is one of the few male members of our female-dominated profession of dietetics!

Glenn has a wonderful knack for picking out the key messages and making them simple and memorable. I've read each of the editions of *Gold Medal Nutrition,* and I've enjoyed every minute of reading. This latest edition is full of the latest information on eating for sporting success. It is broken into sections that tackle a variety of issues related to training and competition—from weight loss to weight gain and

from eating before an event to recovery after. In each section, the science behind sports nutrition is backed up by practical tips on how it applies to the elite athlete or the weekend warrior.

Each topic is covered with bite-sized chunks of useful information. I find myself opening it up to quickly check a fact but then being lured into turning the pages as another box or cartoon grabs my attention. I particularly enjoy the quotes from top athletes and comments from experts.

Now that I know Glenn, I can hear his wit and direct style coming from the pages. I often find myself reading Glenn's work and thinking, *I wish I'd said that.*

Louise Burke, PhD, APD, FACSM
Head of sports nutrition
Australian Institute of Sport

preface

Back in the early 1980s, a colleague of mine suggested we run a marathon. Purchasing the only two books we could find on eating and sport, we set about learning about the best nutrition to complete the distance. They told us that sports drinks were of little value, that fit people could safely lose 4 to 5 per cent of their body weight through sweating before their performance is affected and that athletes probably need less protein than sedentary people because they use protein more efficiently. These books were based on the very little research available at the time. Today, we know differently. There is a huge foundation of research on nutrition and hydration for sports performance, so our advice has greatly improved, yet there is so much more to learn. Now, virtually all elite athletes use the services and advice of sports dietitians and adhere to the nutrition guidelines in this book. Guidelines are the best anyone can offer in a book because athletes differ greatly. Some sweat heavily, whereas others seem to lose very little sweat; as a result, fluid intake advice is going to be different for different athletes. Some will respond to a creatine supplement; others won't. Specific monitoring by a sports dietitian will be invaluable, as will personal experimentation within the guidelines at training sessions.

Gold Medal Nutrition is divided into three parts. Part I discusses the fuel systems used in generating muscle power and gives the principles of good nutrition for healthy body function. It then covers the key aspects of sports nutrition, such as how much carbohydrate, protein, fluid and the key minerals are needed for peak performance, whether for endurance, strength or speed. There has been both confusion and great debate about the athlete's needs for protein, carbohydrate and fluid, and this section makes a big effort to clarify the science.

Part II gets into the practical side of sports nutrition: cooking and the food purchasing habits needed to perform at one's best at training and in competition. Starting with the digestive process, it details the best times to eat meals and snacks so they enhance performance, and how to deal with the all-too-common gastrointestinal distress many athletes experience. You will learn the best nutrition to have before, during and after the event. One chapter discusses the best nutritional supplements for your sport and why some supplements are unlikely to improve your performance.

The final part covers a concern of most athletes—how to control their body fat stores and gain muscle, if necessary. This issue is perhaps the hardest for many athletes. The body seems to have a preconceived view of how much body fat to store. This level of body fat may not be what judges, coaches or the athlete deems ideal. Athletes sometimes must accept a compromise, as getting too lean can weaken performance just as can carrying too much body fat. Increasing muscle mass sounds simple in principle, but it is hard work, and there is a limit to what good nutrition can do. Weight training is going to be the main contributor to an increase in muscle mass.

The first edition of this book, written in 1996, was a small publication for students looking for a simple explanation of the basics of nutrition for sports performance. The book became so popular that second and third editions were produced in 1999 and 2003. Readers said they loved it because, unlike a textbook, it was easy to read and understand, it was fun and it cut straight to the key points. With international interest, this fourth edition has been expanded to cater to all students of the topic. Although it has an Australasian bent, the principles are universal and are based on research conducted throughout the world.

Thanks must go to Mike Bahrke for his faith in this manual. I am most grateful to Chris Drews for her perception, encouragement and wise counsel. Her efforts have greatly improved the book for an international audience. Many of my sports nutrition colleagues from around the globe have given me tips and ideas to place in the manual. The members of Sports Dietitians Australia, the first exclusively sports nutrition professional organisation in the world, have been frequent sources of inspiration.

You are most welcome to send in ideas to include in the next edition. Although many Web sites and books profess to give information on sports nutrition, sadly, very few provide high-quality, unbiased advice. For those readers who want to go deeper and broader than this book allows, please make use of the resources suggested at the back of the book.

part I

Sports Nutrition Principles for Athletes

one

Nutrition and Fuel Systems for Sport

> He must rise at five in the morning, run half a mile at the top of his speed uphill, and then walk six miles at a moderate pace, coming in about seven to breakfast, which should consist of beef steaks or mutton chops, under-done, with stale bread and old beer.
>
> *Captain Robert Barclay Allardice's nutrition advice to long-distance walkers (c. 1810)*

If we asked you to define healthy eating, you would likely give a very acceptable answer: Plenty of fruits and vegetables, whole-grain cereals . . . include lean meats and dairy foods . . . go easy on the cakes and take-aways. Basically, this is correct, but it is so easy to become confused by what we hear from the media and friends and what we read in books and magazines that we often go against our basic instincts. This chapter will help you think about what foods to eat both for health and to get the best out of your body, as well as the nutrients in these foods. We will be going into more detail about the components of food in chapter 2 (protein), chapter 3 (carbohydrate) and chapter 4 (vitamins and minerals).

Good nutrition is quite simple: Eat lots of minimally processed foods such as vegetables, grains, nuts, fruits, lean meats and reduced-fat dairy foods (except Camembert and premium ice cream because they taste the best with the fat left in!). Figure 1.1 shows the healthy eating plate with the major food groups in the proportion needed for good nutrition and to fuel an

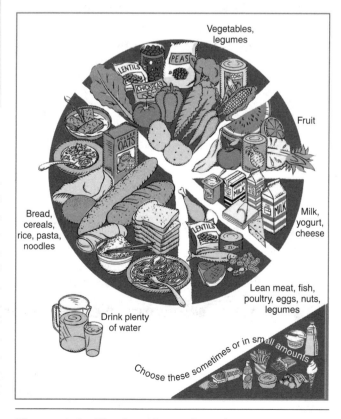

Figure 1.1 The healthy eating plate.
Copyright Commonwealth of Australia. Reproduced by permission.

active body. This healthy eating plate, developed for the Commonwealth Department of Health and Family Services in Australia, is very similar to the food guidelines of most Western nations and is especially suited to athletes and other active people.

Food Groups

Foods are divided into different groups, with each group providing similar essential nutrients. Although nutritionists and sports dietitians vary in how they name the food groups, the underlying science is well established and similar across every reputable source. Table 1.1 lists the minimum serves recommended from each food group for good health.

Fruit, Vegetables and Legumes

This group should make up about a third of what you eat because it plays an essential role in protecting the body from disease now and in the future. This group is the major source of antioxidants and fibre in your diet. These foods also provide appreciable amounts of trace minerals and vitamins. The legumes can be a major protein source for vegetarians (legumes are beans such as kidney beans, lentils and baked beans). This food group is underconsumed by many people in the Western world. Eating more fruit and vegetables can be the single biggest nutritional improvement many people can make. Around the world, 'Eat more fruit and vegetables' campaigns encourage people to eat two serves of fruit (about 300 g [10.5 oz]) and at least 2 cups of vegetables (about 400 g [14 oz]) each day.

One serve of fruit

150 g or 5.3 oz (e.g., 1 medium apple or orange or 2 apricots or 1 cup canned fruit)

One serve of vegetables

1/2 cup cooked vegetables or legumes or 1 cup salad

Breads and Cereals

This group should also comprise around one third of the diet. It includes pasta, rice, bread, breakfast cereals, muesli, and porridge. This group is also a major source of fibre for regularity and general bowel health. Breads and cereals provide some antioxidants, especially in the least processed, whole-grain variety. These foods are your best carbohydrate source; they get broken down to glucose, the main fuel source for active muscles, the liver and the brain.

Some people suggest cutting down or cutting out carbohydrate foods to be healthy and lose weight. In reality, if you do so, you are cutting down on fibre and muscle fuel, making you more prone to tiredness and constipation! High-carbohydrate foods are only likely to make you fat if you are inactive or they come with a lot of added fat, such as pastries and cakes. The least processed grain and cereal foods often provide the most nutrients.

1 serve of breads and cereals

2 slices bread; 1 bread roll; 1 cup of cooked pasta, rice or porridge; 40 g (1.4 oz) breakfast cereal

Milk, Yogurt and Cheese

Dairy foods are your main source of calcium and also provide an appreciable amount of riboflavin and protein. I recommend the lower fat varieties of milk and cheese because they provide less saturated fat and more protein and calcium. Virtually all reduced-fat milks and yogurts have more protein and calcium

Table 1.1 Minimum Serves From Each Food Group for Good Health

Fruit	Vegetables	Breads, cereals	Milk, yogurt, cheese	Meats, legumes	Oil and fat	Treats
2	5	4	2	1	1	1

than the regular versions. If you don't fancy dairy foods, then take some calcium-fortified soy drinks as a substitute. (Make sure soy drinks state they are calcium fortified on the label as there is very little naturally occurring calcium in soy.)

---

1 serve of dairy

1 cup milk; 1 cup calcium-fortified soy drink; 40 g (1.4 oz) cheese; 200 g (7 oz) yogurt

---

Lean Meat, Fish, Poultry, Eggs, Nuts and Legumes

This group of foods is very important in providing protein and essential minerals. Lean meat is a very good source of easy-to-absorb iron and zinc. Fish have gained prominence because the omega-3 fat found in cold-water fish has been strongly linked to a reduced risk of heart attacks. Eggs, nuts and legumes are very important protein sources for many vegetarians. Both nuts and legumes provide fibre and antioxidants so it is no surprise that they appear to lessen the risk of heart disease, some cancers and possibly diabetes.

---

1 serve of meats

100 g (3.5 oz) cooked meat, chicken; 120 g (4.2 oz) cooked fish; 2 eggs; 1/2 cup legumes; 1/3 cup nuts

---

Oil and Fat

Oil and unsaturated margarine provide vitamins D and E and help improve the flavour of many foods. Oil is 100 per cent fat, whereas butter and margarine are around 80 per cent fat. 'Light' margarine may be as low as 40 per cent fat. For most people oil and fat need to be limited as they are high in energy (kilojoules/calories), although athletes can afford a higher fat intake as they are likely to burn it up in training.

Technically, *calories* is often capitalised when referring to kilocalories, but in keeping with common public usage of the term, in this book we will use *calories* to mean kilocalories, even though it is not capitalised. However, kilojoules are never referred to as joules; hence we use the term *kilojoules* for countries that use metric.

---

1 serve of oil and fat

1 Tbsp oil, butter, margarine or 1-1/2 Tbsp reduced-fat spread

---

Treats

OK, these are not really a food group, but they do include a lot of foods that people enjoy as treats or in small amounts in their meals. Some treats provide essential nutrients. Ice cream provides calcium and protein and is a nutritious dessert with canned fruit. Chocolate provides essential vitamins and minerals, along with antioxidants, but being 30 per cent fat, it cannot be eaten in large amounts. Biscuits, cookies, cakes, pastries, pies and take-aways are often high in saturated fat, salt or both; these should be enjoyed, but greatly limited.

---

1 serve of treats

25 g (0.9 oz) chocolate; 40 g (1.4 oz) cake; 30 g (1 oz) crisps; 1 doughnut; one 375 mL (13 oz) can soft drink; 200 mL (7 oz) wine; 400 mL (14 oz) regular beer; 12 hot chips or french fries; 2 cream cookies or biscuits

---

Water

Yes, water is a nutrient, and a most essential one as well. Your body loses fluid each day through exhaled air, urine, sweat, and feces. These losses vary depending on the air temperature and how much sweat you lose each day, but a loss of 1,500 to 3,000 mL of water a day is an average range for active people. You will get your fluid needs from water, tea, coffee, fruit juice, soft drinks, sports drinks and high-water foods such as milk, ice cream, fruits, vegetables and soup. Water requirements are discussed later in the chapter.

Essential Components of Food

Food comprises protein, fat, carbohydrate, fibre, vitamins, minerals and many bio-active compounds such as the antioxidants found mainly in fruits and vegetables. Alcoholic drinks also include alcohol, which is technically a nutrient. We will look at each nutrient in turn.

Protein

Protein is composed of long chains of amino acids (see figure 1.2). Amino acids are the building blocks that make up large protein molecules. The digestive process breaks the protein into groups of one, two or three amino acids, which are then absorbed from the intestine and into the blood to be made into body proteins such as hemoglobin, ferritin, antibodies, enzymes, hair and muscle. Some amino acids must come from food (indispensable or essential amino acids), whereas the body can make the others (dispensable or nonessential).

Protein has many functions in the body:

- Enzymes are forms of protein that enable chemical reactions to take place in the body; they are involved in the digestive breakdown of food via digestive enzymes.

- Cell membranes, tendons and cartilage are composed of structural protein.

- Blood has important forms of protein, such as hemoglobin, which transports oxygen around the blood; transferrin, which transports iron around the body; and albumin, which controls water balance in the cells.

- Antibodies are a specialised form of protein that helps protect us from disease.

- Muscle strength comes from the contractile proteins actin and myosin, which allow muscles to contract and relax in exercise.

Table 1.2   Protein in Food

Good sources	Moderate sources
Meat	Bread
Chicken	Breakfast cereal
Fish	Rice
Seafood	Pasta
Cheese	Oats
Milk	Legumes (e.g.,
Milk powder	baked beans, lentils)
Yogurt	Nuts
Eggs	Seeds

- Skin, nails and hair are made of strong proteins that can cope with the rigours of daily life.

In Western countries, animal foods provide most of the protein. Foods such as meat, chicken, fish, milk, cheese, yogurt and eggs have protein that provide all of the essential amino acids for life (see table 1.2). This is not to discount other valuable sources of protein. About one third of our protein comes from cereal foods (e.g., bread, rice), legumes, fruits and vegetables. Some plant foods will be low in some of the essential amino acids. A combination of plant foods, however, can provide all of the essential amino acids at one meal (complete protein). Some examples are legumes with cereal foods (e.g., beans on toast, lentils with rice) and seeds or nuts with grains (e.g., peanut butter sandwich). In some countries, rice and beans are a major source of complete protein.

If we eat more protein than we require, the excess protein is used as muscle fuel (glucose) during exercise or possibly stored as body fat (but not muscle). Most people, even vegetarians, have no difficulty eating enough protein each day, and protein deficiency is rare in Westernised countries. Those who may be at risk of low protein are those who eat no animal foods (vegans) and those on highly restrictive weight loss diets.

We will discuss amino acids and protein needs, as well as protein supplements, in chapter 2.

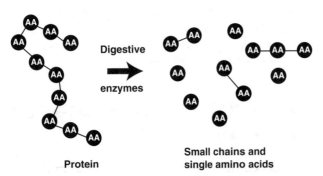

Figure 1.2 Through digestion, chains of amino acids in protein are broken down into small chains or single amino acids. They are then absorbed into the blood to be made into body proteins.

Fat

Although fat in food has received a bad name over the years, fat is actually an essential nutrient. Fat is part of each cell membrane, and in the skin it helps form a barrier against water penetration. Fat is eaten as triglycerides, which consist of a molecule of glycerol bound to three molecules of fatty acids. The two fatty acids essential to life are linoleic acid and linolenic acid. These and other fatty acids can be made into a range of compounds called eicosanoids that control blood clotting, inflammation and immune function.

Fat is found in oils (100 per cent fat), butter and margarine (both about 80 per cent fat); it naturally occurs in oats, whole-grain cereals, nuts, peanut butter, seeds, eggs, avocado, milk, yogurt and cheese. Fat may be added during the manufacture of foods such as cakes, cookies, biscuits and snack foods; or it may be removed, such as in the production of nonfat milk or low-fat yogurt.

For many years there has been a constant message to eat less fat. 'Eat less fat' is an easy take-home message, whereas the more accurate 'Eat less saturated fat' was more difficult to market. Unfortunately, the 'eat less fat' campaigns have given the impression that all fat is bad. More recently we have heard the concept of 'good' and 'bad' fat. The truth has always been that we should be eating less of the 'bad' saturated fat because it causes atherosclerosis (fatty buildup in artery walls) and thrombosis (blood clots). Other types of fat, 'good' unsaturated fat, are unlikely to cause health problems. Table 1.3 shows the types of fat in foods.

Unfortunately, all types of fat eaten in excess are easily converted to body fat. The problem with people in many Western countries, and some athletes, is that they consume too much dietary fat and the excess gets converted to body fat. The more active people are, the less likely this is to happen. Don't see this advice as meaning that you should eat next to no fat because some nutritious foods contain a fair amount of 'healthy' fat, such as nuts and avocado. These foods provide many nutrients and antioxidant chemicals that protect you from disease. It would be crazy to eliminate these from your diet.

Types of Fat

Three main types of fat are found in food: saturated, monounsaturated and polyunsaturated. Another type of fat, called trans fat, also occurs naturally, although too much trans fat in processed fatty foods has been linked to a higher risk of heart disease. Fat is named after the dominant fat type. For example, olive oil is

termed 'monounsaturated' because three quarters of its fat is monounsaturated. Let's take a look at each type of fat found in food.

- **Saturated.** Saturated fat is generally considered the 'bad' fat because of its link to heart disease and some cancers. The term *saturated* is an organic chemistry term meaning that each fatty acid is 'saturated' with the maximum number of hydrogen atoms. The term *saturated*, however, does not mean the food is 'saturated with fat'. Foods high in saturated fat are listed in table 1.3. Saturated fat is generally solid at room temperature and is often added to commercial cakes, biscuits, pastries and take-away foods. To be fair, some take-away franchises are working hard to lower their saturated fat content.

- **Monounsaturated (MU).** This type of fat is viewed quite favourably in health terms and doesn't appear to contribute to future disease. Olive oil, canola oil and the avocado have put MU fat in the spotlight and spawned a range of MU margarines. Nuts, seeds and lean meat also provide some monounsaturated fat. In chemistry terms, *monounsaturated* means that one double bond (hence 'mono') exists between the carbon atoms in the fat, which entails dropping two hydrogen atoms; hence it becomes 'unsaturated' with hydrogen. This is not easy to comprehend unless you have a good knowledge of chemistry, which you will not need to understand the nutrition principles of this book.

- **Polyunsaturated (PU).** This type of fat is considered to be unrelated to poor health. Apart from PU margarines and oils, PU fat also appears in lean meat, nuts and seeds. Oily fish and the fish oils extracted from them are also PU and often referred to as omega-3 fat or marine oils. Some people worry that heating PU fat converts it to saturated fat. Under normal domestic cooking conditions, no unsaturated fat gets converted to saturated fat. In chemistry terms, *polyunsaturated* means that two or more double bonds (hence 'poly') exist between the carbon atoms in the fat, which entails dropping more hydrogen atoms; hence it is 'unsaturated' with hydrogen.

- **Trans fatty acids (TFAs).** TFAs are naturally occurring in ruminant animals, so we find TFAs in beef, lamb, mutton, milk, cheese and yogurt. A TFA is technically an unsaturated fat, but it acts like a saturated fat and could

Table 1.3 Fat in Food

Mainly saturated fat	Mainly unsaturated fat
Cream	Monounsaturated and polyunsaturated margarine
Lard, copha	Monounsaturated and polyunsaturated oil
Butter	Avocado
Cooking margarine	Nuts
Commercial cakes, pastries, cookies and biscuits	Peanut butter
Fatty take-aways	Seeds
French fries, hot chips	Tahini (sesame seed paste)
Hard cheeses, milk, yogurt	Oily fish
Fatty meats, salami, sausages	Lean meats
Snack foods, crisps	

contribute to blocked arteries. Fortunately, the amount of TFAs we get from these foods is not a health problem. Some have been concerned that margarine production resulted in margarines with high TFA levels. Although this remains a problem in some countries, Australia and New Zealand now have virtually eliminated TFAs from table margarine. Check the margarine label as table margarine without TFAs is available in many countries. Hard margarines used in making pastries, cookies and biscuits (also called stick margarine or cooking margarine in supermarkets) are likely to contain TFAs.

How Much Fat Should You Eat?

You are often told that you should eat only 20 to 30 grams of fat a day. Good luck to you. Given that the average man eats more than 100 grams of fat every day, and the average woman, 70 grams of fat, it will take a monumental change and restriction in eating habits to make it down to 20 grams a day. A more realistic daily goal is 40 to 60 grams of fat.

Another common piece of advice given to the public is to avoid any individual food or food product that has more than 10 per cent fat by weight (10 g per 100 g). This means the deletion of avocado, olive oil, nuts, peanut butter, seeds, polyunsaturated margarine and good chocolate, none of which adversely affect the health of your heart or other parts of your body.

Any food that includes oats, chocolate, avocado, nuts and seeds will have a higher fat content; for example, muesli will be 10 per cent fat because of the oats and nuts; peanut butter will be 55 per cent fat, mainly from the peanuts. There is good evidence that they all have nutritional qualities that actually improve your health.

When choosing food, you should consider more than just the fat content. If left on a deserted island, I would choose the peanut butter (55 per cent fat) over jam (0 per cent fat) because it is more nutritious and higher in antioxidant compounds, and the fat is unsaturated. The total fat content of a single food is not the issue; we need to consider the total fat intake of the day, the type of fat and what other nutrients are associated with the fat.

If we take a holistic view of fat in the diet, then the basic points are as follows:

- Eat less saturated fat, as it generally increases the risk of atherosclerosis and thrombosis (e.g., take-aways, cookies, biscuits, pastries). Note: These foods shouldn't be banned, just respected and eaten in sensible amounts.

- Consume most of your fat as unsaturated fat (e.g., lean meats, nuts, seeds, wholegrain cereals, unsaturated oils and margarines).

- Don't eat too much fat, especially if you are inactive, as it is easy to convert to body fat.

Carbohydrate

Without carbohydrate you just cannot perform at your best. Carbohydrate foods provide the crucial energy for muscle contraction and brain function. Some carbohydrate foods also provide fibre necessary for normal bowel function and health, as well as antioxidants that protect the body from heart disease and some cancers. Good sources of carbohydrate are fruits, root vegetables (e.g., potato), rice, pasta, bread, breakfast cereal and legumes. Milk and yogurt have a small amount of carbohydrate in the form of lactose.

Forms of carbohydrate include sugar, of which there are six main types, and starch, of which there are two types. Sugar consists of either a single molecule or two molecules joined together, whereas starch consists of hundreds of sugar molecules joined together. Despite the simple difference, there is so much fantasy, emotion and misinformation about the two.

First let me offer you the basic chemistry behind sugar and starch. Although sugar is often thought of as only table sugar, there are other types of sugar.

Types of Sugar

The main sugars in nature are either a single molecule (monosaccharide) or two molecules joined together (disaccharide) (see figure 1.3). The monosaccharide sugars are as follows:

- Glucose
- Fructose
- Galactose

Galactose is found mainly joined to glucose to form the disaccharide lactose, the sugar found in the milk of almost every mammal.

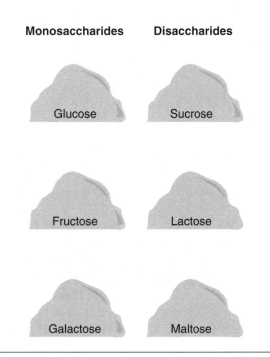

Monosaccharides   **Disaccharides**

Glucose   Sucrose

Fructose   Lactose

Galactose   Maltose

Figure 1.3 The main sugars in food are either monosaccharides (single sugars) or disaccharides (double sugars).

The main disaccharide sugars in nature are as follows:

- Sucrose (glucose + fructose)
- Lactose (glucose + galactose)
- Maltose (glucose + glucose)

The digestive enzymes that break down these disaccharides are called lact*ase*, sucr*ase* and malt*ase*, respectively. (The suffix –*ose* indicates a sugar, and the suffix –*ase* indicates an enzyme; all enzymes are proteins.) About two thirds of the world's adult population lacks the enzyme lactase, meaning that they have a lactose intolerance (*not* an allergy, as some think). A small amount of lactose eaten with a meal usually presents no problem to these people.

Types of Starch

Starchy foods include bread, breakfast cereal, pasta, rice, potato and peas. To the amazement of many, starch is made of hundreds of molecules of just one type of sugar. That sugar is glucose. When starch is digested, it ends up just as glucose, which can then be absorbed. This is important for athletes because this glucose is required to fuel muscle contractions and is needed for brain functioning, allowing the athletes to perform well and think well. Too little carbohydrate means too little glucose for the muscles to work efficiently, which can result in the onset of fatigue. Too little glucose will also affect brain function, meaning that you may not make the best decisions during sport.

Starch is broken down by the digestive enzyme amylase, which breaks down the long chains of glucose to maltose, allowing maltase to break it down further to individual glucose molecules for absorption into the bloodstream. Starch comes in two main forms, amylose and amylopectin, with their different structures affecting the rate at which they are digested. This greatly influences the glycemic index (GI). Carbohydrate and the GI are discussed in greater detail in chapter 3.

Fibre

Since the 1970s fibre has been on the nutrition agenda. Fibre is the undigestable carbohydrate found in plant foods such as grains, vegetables and fruit. It started out as just plain roughage, something to keep you regular. Dr. Denis Burkitt came up with the simple, but unattractive, idea of measuring the weight of human stools (as in waste, not furniture) around the world and linking it to disease. He found that daily stool weight varied from 450 grams in rural Africa to a mere 100 grams in Western societies. His conclusion: More fibre meant more waste and less constipation, hiatus hernia, gallstones, hemorrhoids and possibly bowel cancer. That got everyone adding wheat bran to breakfast cereals. It wasn't tasty, but think of the roughage.

And why all the fuss about fibre? Well, apart from the protection Dr. Burkitt found, it also decreases your risk of high blood cholesterol and helps keep blood sugar levels healthy. That means that eating enough fibre reduces your risk of heart disease and diabetes, so the long-term benefits are substantial. These are all good reasons to enjoy fruits, vegetables, legumes and whole-grain cereals. Fibre is not just one nutrient or component of plant food; rather, it is composed of a range of water-soluble components (pectins, gums and mucilages) and water-insoluble bits (cellulose and hemicellulose). Wheat bran is the most common example

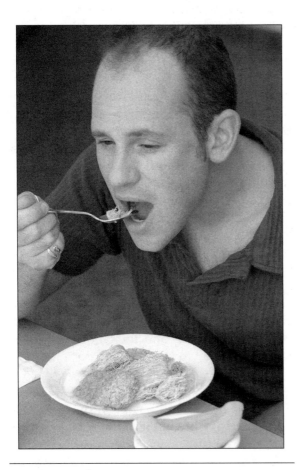

A breakfast of whole-grain cereal, low-fat milk and fruit provides a nutritional start to the day.

of 'insoluble' fibre in our diet, the type of fibre most responsible for keeping us 'regular'.

Some foods are high in 'soluble' fibres, with the best publicised example being oat bran. The year 1988 was when oat bran went crazy. You could get oat bran fibre, oat bran sprinkles, oat bran biscuits and crackers, cereals with added oat bran and, in the United States, oat bran beer. But oat bran broke food's golden rule for success—taste. It tasted awful, so it didn't sell well, although a couple of oat-bran-fortified foods still remain.

It shouldn't be forgotten that oat bran had potential because soluble fibre helps control blood cholesterol and keep it in the healthy range. An easier, tastier and more enjoyable way to get your soluble fibre is through foods such as fruits, rolled oats, muesli and legumes (e.g., kidney beans, baked beans).

Another soluble fibre is psyllium, which is available mainly as a supplement or added to breakfast cereal. Researchers have found that relatively small amounts of psyllium have a modest cholesterol-lowering effect, which could, in turn, reduce heart disease risk.

The latest fibre twist is resistant starch. It's not really a fibre, but it does act a lot like one. Some of the starch you consume has a gel-like consistency and passes through the small intestine without getting digested. It reaches the large intestine and acts similarly to fibre. Some white breads now have added resistant starch. Although not classified as fibre on food labels, resistant starch is providing the benefits of fibre.

Alcohol

The alcohol found in alcoholic drinks is called ethanol, a substance that is toxic to the body. When you hear the word *toxic*, you might start to worry. Don't. It just means that ethanol must be metabolised by the liver as soon as possible, or else it might build up to dangerous levels, which it does when you have had a few too many. Alcohol seems to be safe when consumed in sensible quantities. Indeed, there is very good evidence that having one or two standard drinks a day reduces heart disease risk.

The 'French Paradox' repositioned alcoholic drinks, especially wine, as a 'health' drink. The French Paradox was the observation that the French eat as much artery-clogging saturated fat as we do, yet have half the heart disease. It was believed that the answer lay in the antioxidants found in red wine. These are compounds that stop blood cholesterol from converting to its most damaging form, and stop the DNA in normal cells from mutating into cancer cells. In other words, these are very clever chemicals, indeed.

Of course, there were some things you weren't told about the French Paradox. Apart from enjoying more wine, the French also eat more, and a greater range of, fruits and vegetables than we do. Fruits and vegetables are an abundant source of antioxidants and are proven to reduce heart disease. This suggests that other aspects of the French lifestyle are protecting against heart disease. However, alcohol could be playing its part on its own accord. Alcohol reduces the chance of blood clots (thrombosis) forming in the blood vessels and blocking blood flow. That makes beer and spirits in sensible amounts candidates for a heart healthy award too.

Research suggests a maximum of three standard drinks a day for long-term health in men. Two standard drinks daily is the maximum recommended for nonpregnant women. Most health authorities recommend that pregnant women consume no alcohol because it can affect fetal development.

Remember that alcohol is a diuretic, meaning that it can make you pass a greater volume of fluid (as urine) than you take in from the alcoholic drinks, possibly leading to dehydration. For this reason, you will need more nonalcoholic fluids in your diet when drinking alcohol.

Water

Around 60 per cent of your total body weight is water. That's about 40 litres (10.5 gal) of water in a 70-kilogram (154 lb) person. Water makes up most of your blood, your urine and your sweat and is the main component of each body cell. Water is crucial to the regulation of body temperature to prevent overheating, which will quickly impair sports performance. Too little water in the body is called dehydration and can lead to thermal stress and heatstroke. Fluid replacement is discussed in more detail in chapter 5.

I've heard many times—and no doubt you have too—that you should drink six to eight glasses of water each day. If this statement is based on human physiology, then it is flawed from the start. I originally thought that the claim was based on the physiology textbooks that state that the average human produces 1,500 mL of urine each day. If a glass is 200 to 250 mL (7 to 8 oz), then that means that you produce the equivalent of six to eight glasses of urine a day. It makes logical sense that you

Standard Drinks

Alcoholic drinks are measured as standard drinks. One standard drink is any of the following:

- 285 mL (10 oz) full-strength beer (5 per cent alcohol)
- Two 285 mL (10 oz) reduced-alcohol beer (2.5 per cent alcohol)
- 100 mL (3 oz) wine
- 60 mL (2 oz) port, sherry
- 30 mL (1 nip) spirits

One standard drink provides 10 grams of alcohol; in the United Kingdom one alcohol unit provides 8 grams of alcohol (see also chapter 5 on fluids).

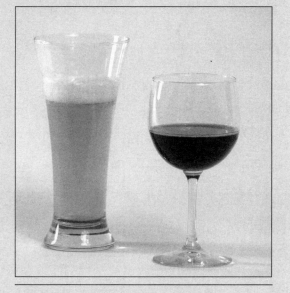

A standard drink is 285 mL (10 oz) of full-strength beer or 100 mL (3 oz) of wine.

should drink enough water to replace urine losses, but this may not be as logical as it seems. There are other water losses from the body via the skin (500 mL [17 oz]—more if you sweat through exercise or in hot conditions), exhalation (350 mL [12 oz]) and in feces (150 mL [5 oz]). Does that mean you need more than eight glasses of water a day?

A lot of the 'solid' foods you eat contain appreciable amounts of water. Vegetables and fruits are around 90 per cent water, as is milk, fruit juice and soft drinks. Cooked meats and fish are over 50 per cent water, and breads are about one third water (see table 1.4). So, a meat and salad sandwich will provide 160 mL (5 oz) of water. Add a piece of fruit and a glass of milk, and you will have around 470 mL (16 oz)

Table 1.4 Approximate Water Content of Some Foods

Food	Water content
Soft drink, 200 mL (7 oz)	185 mL (6 oz)
Fruit juice, 200 mL (7 oz)	185 mL (6 oz)
Milk, 200 mL (7 oz)	180 mL (6 oz)
Fruit salad, 200 g (7 oz)	170 mL (6 oz)
Yogurt, 200 g (7 oz)	160 mL (5 oz)
Apple, 150 g (5.3 oz)	130 mL (4 oz)
Tomato, 100 g (3.5 oz)	93 mL (3 oz)
Broccoli, 100 g (3.5 oz)	90 mL (3 oz)
Potato salad, 100 g (3.5 oz)	75 mL (2.5 oz)
Baked beans, 100 g (3.5 oz)	75 mL (2.5 oz)
Avocado, 100 g (3.5 oz)	73 mL (2.5 oz)
Ham, 100 g (3.5 oz)	70 mL (2.5 oz)
Chicken, 100 g (3.5 oz)	50 mL (2 oz)
Egg, boiled, 50 g (1.8 oz)	35 mL (1 oz)
Cheddar cheese, 30 g (1 oz)	10 mL (1/3 oz)
Bread, 1 slice	10 mL (1/3 oz)
Breakfast cereal, 100 g (3.5 oz)	5 mL (1/6 oz)
Peanuts, raw, 100 g (3.5 oz)	5 mL (1/6 oz)
Vegetable oil, 1 Tbsp	0 mL

of water. As you can see, water doesn't have to be your only source of water.

Thirst is not a good indication of fluid needs when exercising and working under hot conditions. Under those conditions it is wise to drink at the rate of 1 litre (1 qt) per hour to minimise your risk of dehydration. Under most other conditions, your thirst response works wonderfully well, as you would expect after years of human evolution, mostly in a hot environment.

You should drink as much fluid as you need to keep hydrated. In most cases, this is the amount of fluid that will produce pale urine about five or six times a day. On a hot day, that might be 3 litres or more; on a cool winter's day, that might be only four cups of tea or coffee, with your food providing the rest of your fluid needs. That's right, even tea and coffee are fluid sources to the body (see the section on diuretics in chapter 5).

Vitamins

Vitamins are often divided into water-soluble and fat-soluble types. The water-soluble ones are vitamin C and the B group vitamins (thiamin, riboflavin, niacin, pyridoxine, biotin, pantothenic acid, folate and vitamin B_{12}). The fat-soluble ones are vitamins A, D, E and K. Although most people will get their vitamin requirements by eating well, about half of all athletes take a vitamin supplement.

The vitamin folate has received a lot of publicity. It is often given as a supplement to women just before, and during, pregnancy to reduce the risk of spinal deformities in the baby. Accumulating evidence suggests that a high level of homocysteine in the blood dramatically increases the risk of heart disease, a major killer of men and women. (Homocysteine is similar to an amino acid and occurs naturally in the body.) Adequate folate in the diet lowers elevated homocysteine levels and reduces the risk of a heart attack. Folate also appears to reduce cancer and dementia risk too. The amount of folate recommended is 400 micrograms a day (see table 1.5). (See also the discussion of vitamins in sport in chapter 4.)

Minerals

Getting too few minerals is not a common problem for most men because their needs are usually met by food intake (see table 1.6). For

Table 1.5   Vitamins in Food

Vitamin	Good food sources	Australia and New Zealand recommended daily needs (NRV)	United States and Canada recommended daily needs (DRI)	UK recommended daily needs (RNI)
Thiamin	Whole grains, nuts, legumes, bread, fortified breakfast cereals, meat, yeast extract	1.1 mg women 1.2 mg men	1.1 mg women 1.2 mg men	0.8 mg women 1.0 mg men
Riboflavin	Milk, yogurt, yeast extracts, fortified breakfast cereals, almonds, meat	1.1 mg women 1.3 mg men	1.1 mg women 1.3 mg men	1.1 mg women 1.3 mg men
Niacin	Meat, poultry, fish, yeast extracts, peanuts, legumes, whole-grain bread	14 mg women 16 mg men	14 mg women 16 mg men	13 mg women 17 mg men
Vitamin B_6 Pyridoxine	Meats, whole grains, vegetables, nuts	1.3 mg	1.3 mg	1.2 mg women 1.4 mg men
Biotin	Widely distributed in food	Adequate intake: 25 mcg women 30 mcg men	Adequate intake: 30 mcg women 30 mcg men	N/A
Pantothenic acid	Widely distributed in whole foods	Adequate intake: 4 mg women 6 mg men	Adequate intake: 5 mg women 5 mg men	N/A
Folate	Fruit, avocado, vegetables (especially green leafy), lentils, folate-fortified breakfast cereals, yeast extract	400 mcg 600 mcg pregnancy	400 mcg 600 mcg pregnancy	200 mcg 260 mcg pregnancy
Vitamin B_{12}	Fish, meats, egg, milk, cheese, yogurt	2.4 mcg	2.4 mcg	1.5 mcg
C	Fruit, fruit juice, canned fruit, vegetables	45 mg	75 mg women 90 mg men	40 mg
A	Milk, butter, margarine, cheese, egg, liver; yellow and orange fruits and vegetables for beta-carotene	700 mcg women 900 mcg men	700 mcg women 900 mcg men	600 mcg women 700 mcg men
D	Oily fish, margarine, liver, cheese, action of sunlight on skin	Adequate intake: 5–10 mcg (higher amount in over 50 yr)	Adequate intake: 5–10 mcg (higher amount in over 50 yr)	N/A
E	Wheat germ, nuts, avocado, margarine, meat, poultry, fish	Adequate intake: 7 mg women 10 mg men	15 mg women 15 mg men	N/A
K	Green leafy vegetables, liver, legumes	Adequate intake: 60 mcg women 70 mcg men	Adequate intake: 90 mcg women 120 mcg men	N/A

Note: The figures given represent the amount that will provide the requirements for virtually everyone and are not minimum requirements. NRV = nutrient reference value; DRI = dietary reference intake; RNI = reference nutrient intake; mg = milligrams; mcg = micrograms; N/A = not available.

Adequate intake: No recommended daily requirement has been established. The level at which intake should be adequate for normal body function has been determined from the best available data.

Table 1.6　Minerals in Food

Mineral	Good food sources	Australia and New Zealand recommended daily needs (NRV)	United States and Canada recommended daily needs (DRI)	UK recommended daily needs (RNI)
Iron	Meats, iron-fortified foods (e.g., breakfast cereals and Milo)	8 mg men 18 mg women <50 yr 8 mg women >50 yr	8 mg men 18 mg women <50 yr 8 mg women >50 yr	8.7 mg men 14.8 mg women <50 yr 8.7 mg women >50 yr
Calcium	Milks, yogurt, cheese, calcium-fortified soy milk and drinks, ice cream, canned fish with soft edible bones, milk chocolate	1,000 mg 1,300 mg women >50 yr 1,300 mg men >70 yr	1,000 mg 1,200 mg women >50 yr 1,200 mg men >50 yr	700 mg 700 mg women >50 yr 700 mg men >50 yr
Zinc	Meats, seafood, nuts, milk, cheese	8 mg women 14 mg men	8 mg women 11 mg men	7 mg women 9.5 mg men
Chromium	Nuts, meat, fruit, vegetables, cheese, egg	Adequate intake: 25 mcg women 35 mcg men	Adequate intake: 25 mcg women 35 mcg men	N/A
Copper	Seafood, nuts, legumes, chocolate	Adequate intake: 1.2 mg women 1.7 mg men	0.9 mg women 0.9 mg men	1.2 mg women 1.2 mg men
Selenium	Fish, meats, cereals, grains	55 mcg women 65 mcg men	55 mcg women 55 mcg men	60 mcg women 75 mcg men
Iodine	Seafood	150 mcg	150 mcg	140 mcg
Magnesium	Green vegetables, nuts, legumes, bread	320 mg women 420 mg men	320 mg women 420 mg men	270 mg women 300 mg men
Sodium	Many processed foods contain added salt or sodium	Adequate intake: 460–920 mg Maximum: 1,600 mg	Maximum: 2,400 mg	Maximum: 1,600 mg
Potassium	Fruit, vegetables	Adequate intake: 4,700 mg	Minimum: 2,000 mg	3,500 mg

Note: The figures given represent the amount that will provide the requirements for virtually everyone and are not minimum requirements. NRV = nutrient reference value; DRI = dietary reference intake; RNI = reference nutrient intake; mg = milligrams; mcg = micrograms; N/A = not available.

Adequate intake: No recommended daily requirement has been established. The level at which intake should be adequate for normal body function has been determined from the best available data.

example, iron deficiency anemia is not common in men because they can usually get enough iron through eating lean meat and iron-fortified breakfast cereals alone. Inadequate mineral intake, especially of iron, calcium and zinc, is of concern to some women, with over half of women getting less than the recommended intake of these minerals. (See chapter 4 for more on iron and calcium.) One mineral of concern is sodium, which is most commonly found in the form of sodium chloride (salt). Too much salt is not good for long-term health and may contribute to bone loss and high blood pressure. I recommend that you choose low-salt or reduced-salt versions of processed foods and that you wean yourself from the taste of salty foods.

Note that some salty foods don't taste salty. Cornflakes don't taste salty, yet they contain 800 milligrams of sodium per 100 grams. Compare that to salty potato crisps at 600 milligrams per 100 grams. A breakfast cereal with more than 400 milligrams of sodium per 100 grams is considered quite high in salt. A low-salt food has less than 120 milligrams of sodium per 100 grams.

Vitamin and Mineral Supplements

Sometimes your doctor may recommend that you take a vitamin or mineral supplement based on an established deficiency. Some researchers suggest that you take a multivitamin supplement after the age of 65 years as your body may have a reduced ability to absorb nutrients. These supplements can also be very useful on other occasions, such as when you travel overseas and cannot be sure you are eating well. If you are bush walking or camping for weeks at a time, then consider a supplement to complement the limited range of foods you might take with you. Other than that, it is pretty much an individual decision.

Don't expect wonderful results from taking a vitamin supplement. Some people take them in the hope that they will give them vitality and diffuse the general fatigue they suffer, when a change of job or relationship, or improving their diet, would have had a far better outcome. Vitamin supplements will not compensate for poor nutrition choices. The evidence suggests that eating fruits and vegetables and being active provide far more health benefits than taking a supplement does. If you do choose a supplement, make sure it provides only 50 to 100 per cent of your daily needs (see tables 1.5 and 1.6). More than this is generally excreted in the urine (hence the iridescent glow-in-the-dark stream!).

Antioxidants

Without oxygen you would die quickly. Oxygen keeps you alive, but it is also slowly killing you because oxygen is toxic over a lifetime. Inhaling air naturally produces harmful free radicals that cause a slow rusting, or aging, of the body. The rusting is properly termed oxidation and

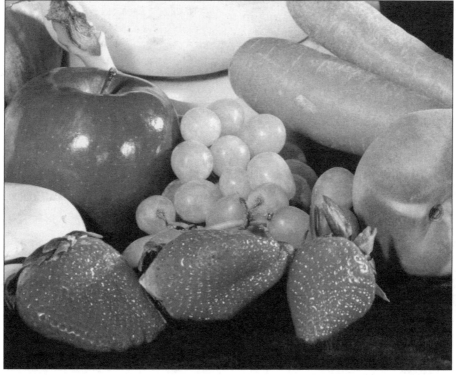

© Art Explosion

Eat plenty of fruits and vegetables to reap the benefits of fibre, vitamins, minerals and antioxidants. Two serves of fruit and five serves of vegetables is considered a healthy baseline intake.

is the reason we slowly age. To slow down the oxidation process, antioxidation chemicals are needed, hence the term 'antioxidants'.

There is now evidence that the harm caused by oxygen can accumulate and contribute to diseases such as heart disease and cancer and other health problems such as eye cataracts and rheumatoid arthritis. The free radicals may cause damage to DNA molecules so that new body cells mutate and become cancer cells. Free radical damage to blood cholesterol can make the cholesterol far more damaging to your artery lining than previously realised. (Note: Free radicals are not always harmful. Clever blood cells called phagocytes produce free radicals to kill disease-causing microbes.)

Fortunately, through evolution, humans have devised ways to minimise the toxic damage of oxygen. The body produces special antioxidant enzymes to soak up free radicals. They have names such as glutathione, catalase and superoxide dismutase. Certain minerals can help those enzymes do their job efficiently, such as selenium, copper, manganese and zinc. The antioxidants we eat as food are a bonus that helps reduce our chance of heart disease and some cancers.

Vitamins can also act as antioxidants, the best known being vitamin C, vitamin E and beta-carotene. More recently, the spotlight has been on non-nutrient antioxidants found in food, such as phenols, flavonoids and carotenoids other than beta-carotene. Phenols have been found in red wine, tea and chocolate and are widely distributed in the plant kingdom. If you don't like wine, grape juice has similar antioxidants as red wine.

It is estimated that at least 5,000 compounds in foods have antioxidant properties, many of them being in fruits and vegetables. For example, there are over 500 different carotenoids in food. Scientists uniformly agree that the highest consumers of fruits and vegetables are the least likely to get heart disease or cancer.

Manufacturers add antioxidants to foods to stop them from deteriorating and 'going off', hence giving them a longer shelf life. Many foods containing fat and oil have added antioxidants to protect against rancidity as a result of exposure to oxygen. Even a small amount of rancid fat will ruin the flavour and smell of a food. Sulphur dioxide is added to dried apricots to stop the discolouration caused by

oxygen. Vacuum sealing of foods also helps keep the food away from oxygen.

Fuel Systems

We have discussed foods and nutrients and the amounts you need for good health. Before we cover specific nutrient needs in fitness and sport, we will explore how the body produces the energy you need for exercise. Many nutrients are involved in energy production during exercise. The two major fuels for energy are fat and carbohydrate. The next section will look at how we burn energy.

Your body is perfectly designed to move by a coordinated series of muscle contractions. When your brain tells your body to move, nerve signals trigger a powerful release of muscle energy through a special molecule called adenosine triphosphate (ATP). ATP is a high-energy molecule that, when its phosphate bonds snap apart, provides the energy for muscle contraction and away you go. ATP is generated in mitochondria, the powerhouses of each body cell, from the energy you eat as food. Each muscle cell contains thousands of mitochondria. Three systems in the body create the ATP energy required for physical activity.

ATP-CP System

The ATP-CP system provides enough energy for a five- or six-second sprint or other rapid muscle contraction such as lifting weights. Creatine phosphate (CP) is a high-energy molecule that can deliver its energy to manufacture ATP very quickly. A resting muscle has about four times more CP than ATP. During muscle contraction the CP transfers its energy to ATP production (see figure 1.4), but the CP reserves are drained quite quickly. Stocks of CP in the

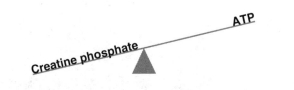

Figure 1.4 Creatine phosphate transfers its energy to produce more ATP for quick bursts of muscle contraction, leading to a drop in creatine phosphate and a rapid rise in ATP.

muscles are remade during the next rest period between sprints.

Many strength and sprint athletes now take creatine supplements to make sure they have maximum creatine phosphate levels in their muscles. (See chapter 8 for more on creatine.) No oxygen is required for this system to work, so you don't need to inhale air during a very short sprint. Because no oxygen is required, it is called anaerobic ('without oxygen') exercise.

Glycolytic System

The glycolytic system is most important for high-power efforts lasting up to two minutes. When CP levels are low, the muscles turn to glucose for rapid production of ATP, again with little requirement for oxygen. This anaerobic system generates only two ATP molecules from each glucose molecule (see figure 1.5).

Unfortunately, lactic acid is a by-product of the glycolytic system, and too much lactic acid will cause muscle fatigue. The muscle avoids acid fatigue by switching to a third system that requires oxygen, the aerobic system. As exercise intensity rises, the body relies more on the glycolytic system fueled by glucose. When the intensity is lower (e.g., during walking or jogging), the body prefers the aerobic system that uses both fat and glucose for muscle fuel.

Aerobic System

The word *aerobic* is a combination of the Greek words *aero* (air) and *bios* (life). As the name implies, plenty of oxygen is required for this system to work efficiently. This system is most important in any exercise that lasts longer than two minutes. It is also known as oxidative phosphorylation and uses both glucose and fat as its fuel source. All this action takes place in the

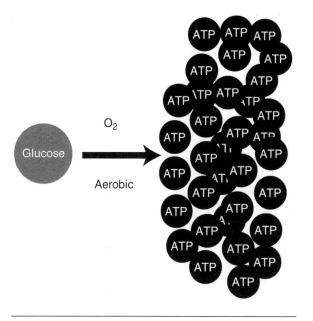

Figure 1.6 While you are exercising at low to medium intensity, one glucose molecule is metabolised to produce an extra 34 ATP molecules, for a total of 36.

mitochondria, which are abundant in muscle cells and in the cardiac cells of the heart.

The inhaled oxygen helps the muscles produce an extra 34 ATP molecules from one glucose molecule, making a total of 36 ATPs compared to only two without oxygen (see figure 1.6). Glucose is the most efficient fuel as it produces more ATP with each breath than does fat or protein. Your major source of glucose is the carbohydrate (sugar and starch) in your diet.

However, body stores of glucose are limited compared to body stores of fat. Endurance training helps muscles use fat more efficiently as a fuel, thereby making fewer demands on glucose and improving endurance. Amino acids from protein are sometimes used as a fuel, mainly near the end of endurance sports when glucose stores are low. Note: The three energy systems operate at the same time, but their relative contribution varies with the intensity and duration of the sport.

Maximum Fuel Stores

Glucose is stored in the muscles as long chains that form the giant molecule called glycogen. Hence, we refer to glycogen as the primary muscle fuel. Glycogen is specially structured

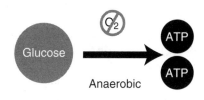

Figure 1.5 In the anaerobic glycolytic system, the glucose molecule produces two ATP molecules.

to break down quickly to glucose as required by the muscles.

Carbohydrate in food is digested, absorbed into the blood and transported to muscles to be converted to glycogen (see figure 1.7). Glycogen is stored in both your muscles and your liver. The average fit 70-kilogram (154 lb) person will have 165 kilojoules (40 calories) of glucose in the blood and store around 1,100 kilojoules (260 calories) of glycogen in the liver and 5,900 kilojoules (1,400 calories) of glycogen in the muscles. If you want to train and compete efficiently, you need a full fuel tank of glycogen every time you exercise.

During exercise the body will burn a mixture of fat and glycogen, but glycogen is the fuel that will run out the quickest. The glycogen molecule releases glucose units as they are needed by the muscle. Glucose is the preferred muscle fuel, especially as exercise intensity increases. During high-intensity exercise, glycogen is used at a very fast rate and may become

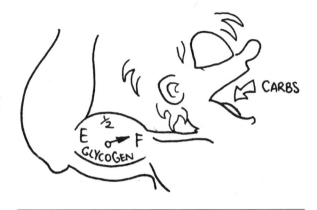

Carbohydrate in food will replenish the glycogen fuel tank in working muscles.

depleted after 30 to 45 minutes, yet it may last for 180 minutes in a brisk walk.

At lower intensity (e.g., walking, recovery sessions) both body fat and glycogen are used as fuel. Even a slim person will carry 250,000 kilojoules (about 60,000 calories) or more of fat, so fat fuel never runs out. (Theoretically, 250,000 kilojoules is enough energy to run 1,000 km or 620 miles!) Glycogen is the 'limiting' fuel; in other words, there is a limit to how much the body can store. In hot weather glycogen may be burned at a faster rate than in cooler temperatures.

Maintaining Fuel Levels

Muscle glycogen levels vary among people. A trained athlete will have more muscle glycogen than will someone doing little activity. Fit people aim to keep muscle glycogen levels as high as possible so they can train effectively for long periods and recover quickly. Or they may just want to be able to walk longer or just get through a day's work.

Glycogen is stored mainly in the active muscles; hence, cyclists and runners will preferentially store, and then use up, the glycogen in their leg muscles. Swimmers will store lots of glycogen in their arm and leg muscles. Unfortunately, if your leg muscles run out of glycogen, you can't bring in more from your arms and vice versa.

When muscle glycogen levels are low and blood glucose levels start to drop, it is called 'hitting the wall' (cyclists, strangely, call this 'bonking'), an altogether unsavoury feeling of extreme fatigue, dizziness and hunger.

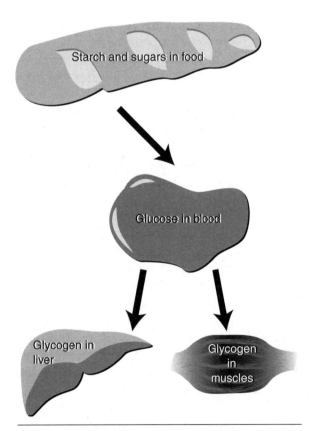

Figure 1.7 Starches and sugars in food become glucose in the blood or are stored as glycogen in the muscles and liver. Glycogen then breaks down to glucose as required by the body.

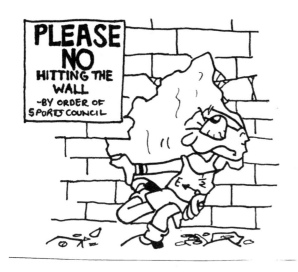

If you 'hit the wall,' evaluate whether you ate enough carbohydrate.

This feeling can be partially reversed by consuming some quick-to-absorb carbohydrate, such as a sports drink or soft confectionery (candy). If you ever do 'hit the wall', evaluate your eating habits in the 24 hours before the event and your nutrition during the event. There is a good chance you didn't consume enough carbohydrate before or during the event.

Glycogen Power

In time-and-motion analyses of football (soccer) games, players travel 9 to 12 kilometres (6 to 7 miles) in 90 minutes of play. Players with plenty of glycogen travelled 12 kilometres, with only a quarter (3 km) of that at a walk. Players with low glycogen stores travelled only 9.5 kilometres and about half (4.7 km) of that was at a walk. Researchers concluded that 'the more glycogen, the further and faster the player ran' (Kirkendall 1993, p. 1372).

Liver glycogen is the main source of blood glucose, and overnight your liver glycogen can drop by two thirds. This is a key reason you should eat something before an event, especially after an overnight fast (i.e., sleep-

ing). There should be enough fuel for an early morning training session of 60 minutes, however, provided you ate enough carbohydrate the night before.

When you run out of muscle glycogen, your muscles begin to take up more glucose from your blood (see figure 1.8). At this point your liver comes to the rescue. The hormone glucagon races off to the liver and asks the liver to now convert its glycogen to glucose and pump it into the blood. Taking a sports drink will also help keep blood glucose levels up during long events.

When liver glycogen levels run low, the adrenal gland releases the hormone cortisol. Cortisol tells some of the muscle protein to break down to amino acids, which then go to the liver to be made into glucose and released into the blood. You can see why it's smart to have lots of glycogen in your muscles and liver before you start—it means you won't burn up muscle protein.

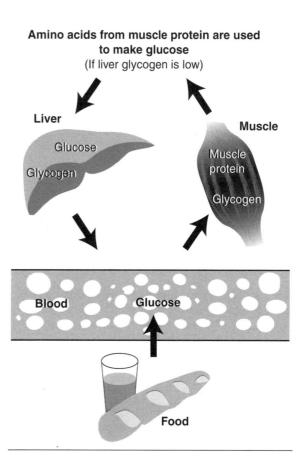

Figure 1.8 The glucose cycle. Carbohydrate-containing food and drinks are absorbed as glucose into the blood. From there, glucose is transported to the muscles and liver to be stored as glycogen.

FINAL SCORE

- Protein is plentiful in most people's diets. Most people eat more than they need, unless the diet is highly restricted.

- Fat is essential to health. It is mainly saturated fat that should be limited as it can be harmful to overall health.

- If you are active and relatively lean, you don't have to severely limit your unsaturated fat intake.

- Forms of carbohydrate include both sugar, of which there are six common types in nature (glucose, fructose, galactose, sucrose, lactose and maltose), and starch, of which there are two main types (amylose and amylopectin).

- Sugars are a normal part of the diet. They are not harmful, except when you eat so much added-sugar foods that they displace other nutritious foods.

- Some sugar-containing foods are very nutritious, such as fruits, milk, yogurt, soy drinks and chocolate.

- Starches are long chains of glucose molecules. Starchy foods generally also provide essential minerals, vitamins, antioxidants and fibre.

- Fibre is found only in plant foods. If you eat plenty of fruits, vegetables and whole-grain cereals, you will likely be getting enough fibre for health.

- Plant foods are very protective against future disease because of their high levels of essential nutrients, fibre and antioxidants.

- The first five or six seconds of a sprint activity relies on creatine phosphate to activate the ATP.

- High-intensity exercise relies mainly on glucose for energy.

- Lower-intensity activity relies on the aerobic system, which uses both fat and glucose as fuels.

- Glycogen is the rate-limiting fuel. When glycogen stores are low, fatigue results. For greatest endurance, a high-carbohydrate diet is required.

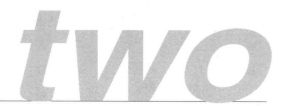

Protein for Growth and Maintenance

Protein requirements are slightly increased in highly active people. . . . These recommended protein intakes can generally be met through diet alone, without the use of protein or amino acid supplements, if energy intake is adequate to maintain body weight.

American College of Sports Medicine (2000)

In the 6th century BC, the Greek athlete Milo of Crotonia won wrestling gold in six Olympic games and was recognised as one of the world's strongest men. He may have developed the first progressive resistance exercise program by lifting a calf daily. As the calf grew, Milo continued to lift it, and his muscles became stronger. When the calf was four years old, Milo had her for dinner. It was common for him to eat 5 to 8 kilograms (11 to 18 pounds) of meat a day. Was it Milo who sparked the great protein debate?

The popular view of most athletes today is that muscles, being made of protein, will get bigger the more protein they eat. Lean steaks, skinless chicken, amino acids and protein powders attract those in search of the larger latissimus, the bigger biceps, and the gargantuan gastrocnemius. Do we know how much protein an athlete needs? Let's take a look at the science.

What Are Proteins and Amino Acids?

Protein is composed of long chains of amino acids. The amino acids that the body can make are called nonessential amino acids. Eight amino acids, called essential amino acids, can't be made by the body and must be provided by foods (see table 2.1). (Scientists now use the terms *indispensable* and *dispensable* for essential and nonessential amino acids, respectively, but as the latter two terms are better known and understood, we will continue using them.)

High-protein foods of animal origin such as meat, chicken, fish, milk, cheese, yogurt and eggs will provide all of the essential amino acids. This is not to discount other valuable sources of protein from plant foods. About one third of our protein comes from cereal foods (e.g., bread, rice), legumes, fruits and vegetables.

Some plant foods will be low in some of the essential amino acids. A combination of plant foods can provide all the essential amino acids at the one meal, with one food compensating for a low level of an essential amino acid in another food. For example, grains can be low in the essential amino acid lysine, whereas legumes may be low in the essential amino acid methionine. By combining legumes with cereal

Table 2.1   Amino Acids

Essential amino acids	Nonessential amino acids
Isoleucine	Alanine
Leucine	Arginine
Lysine	Asparagine
Methionine	Aspartic acid
Phenylalanine	Cystine (cysteine)
Threonine	Glutamic acid
Tryptophan	Glutamine
Valine	Glycine
	Histidine
	Hydroxyproline
	Hydroxyglycine
	Proline
	Serine
	Taurine
	Tyrosine

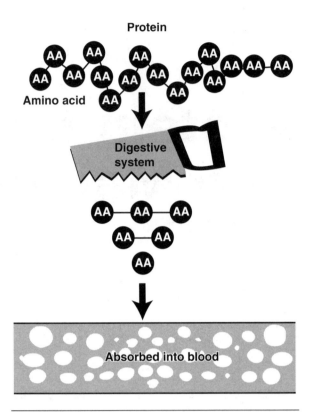

Figure 2.1   Long chains of amino acids in protein are broken down by digestive enzymes into lengths of one, two or three amino acids for absorption into the blood.

foods (e.g., beans on toast, lentils with rice) and seeds or nuts with grains (e.g., peanut butter sandwich), the body gets adequate amounts of both amino acids from a meal.

Many believe that all the essential amino acids need to be eaten at each meal, but this is not necessary. If a person consumes a range of protein foods throughout the day, enough amino acids will be circulating in the body from which it can select the essential amino acids it needs. As long as the diet provides the minimum essential amino acids over 24 hours, there is no risk of a protein deficiency. This is quite simple for ovo-lacto vegetarians because they eat eggs, milk, cheese and yogurt, all containing adequate amounts of essential amino acids. Only the vegan, who eats no animal foods, is at risk of too little protein. Soy milk, nuts, legumes and grains can provide sufficient protein for vegans, although I do suggest that vegan athletes consult a sports dietitian to ensure they are getting adequate nutrition.

Getting enough protein each day is not difficult, and virtually all athletes and active people will get what they need from regular meals and snacks.

Protein Digestion: From Mouth to Blood

A small amount of the protein we eat is digested in the stomach, but the majority is digested in the small intestine. Here the protein is broken down into smaller chains of amino acids (peptides) by digestive enzymes. The

end results of digestion are single amino acids and small peptides of two or three amino acids joined together as shown in figure 2.1. These are then absorbed from the intestine and into the blood to be made into body proteins such as hemoglobin, ferritin, antibodies, enzymes, hair and muscle.

Amino acids in the form of small peptides are more rapidly and efficiently absorbed than are single amino acids (commonly called 'free form' amino acids) because they are absorbed through different pathways. This is a fact we have known since 1962, yet the notion that 'free form' amino acids are the best way to get amino acids is still widely promoted. The most efficient way to take your amino acids is as food protein, preferably a low-fat version such as nonfat milk or chicken breast.

Protein Needs of Athletes

The value of protein to athletes has been debated for over 100 years in the scientific literature. In the early 1900s protein was considered essential for muscle strength and the most important fuel for exercise. In the 1970s the scientific opinion was that the protein needs of athletes were the same as those of sedentary people. Now there is universal agreement that active people, especially athletes, require more protein than sedentary people do.

There is still a lot of debate over the protein needs of different athletes under various sporting conditions. Although I have given a table of protein requirements (see table 2.2), please be aware that these are 'guidelines of best fit' at the time of writing. This advice will be refined with further research. Indeed, some research hints that athletes don't need as much protein as indicated in table 2.2. For example, a 65-kilogram (143 lb) female endurance athlete will require about 66 grams of protein daily. This is calculated by multiplying 65 by 1.2 grams per kilogram of body weight (78) and then reducing this figure by 15 per cent (78 × 0.85 = 66 grams). If you are carrying excess body fat, then base your protein requirements on your ideal weight. If you are already well muscled and have normal body fat levels, then calculate your protein needs on your current weight.

During exercise the body relies mainly on muscle glycogen, liver glycogen and fat stores for fuel. However, athletes doing high-intensity training or endurance training for more than an hour may use some protein for muscle fuel, especially if glycogen stores are low. In other words, if too little carbohydrate is consumed, muscle protein and amino acids in the blood are converted to glucose to be used as muscle fuel. Weight training uses mainly carbohydrate as a fuel during intense sets. Protein is also needed for muscle growth and repair after resistance training, intense exercise or endurance training.

Protein may account for 5 to 10 per cent of the energy men use in endurance training. This is normally less in women, who make better use of fat as a fuel and are therefore better fat burners than men are. A greater amount of protein is used as muscle fuel if muscle glycogen stores are low. For this reason, be sure to pump your glycogen stores with plenty of carbohydrate before sport to stop your body from using protein as fuel. Note: High-carbohydrate foods are generally cheaper than protein foods, so fuelling your body right could save you money.

How Much Protein Do You Need?

Sports nutrition experts agree that the healthy-eating ideals covered so far in this book will provide the needs of virtually all athletes.

Table 2.2 Recommended Daily Intake of Protein

Type of person	grams/kg IBW[a]/day	75 kg man	65 kg woman[b]
Adults, nonathletes	0.8	60	52
Elite endurance athletes	1.6	120	88
Endurance athletes	1.2–1.4	90–105	66–77
Power sports	1.4–1.7	105–127	77–94
Strength athletes (early training)	1.5–1.7	112–127	83–94
Strength athletes (steady state)	1.0–1.2	75–90	55–66
Recreational athletes	1.0	75	55
Actual daily intake of protein			
Average adult eats	1.0–1.5		
Average female athlete eats	1.0–2.8		
Average male athlete eats	1.5–4.0		

[a]IBW = ideal body weight.

[b]Female athletes require about 15% less protein than male athletes.

Data sources include Nutrient Reference Values for Australia and New Zealand 2004; Lemon, P.W.R. 1998. Effects of exercise on dietary protein requirements. *International Journal of Sport Nutrition* 8:426-447; Tarnopolsky, M. 2000. *Clinical Sports Nutrition.* New York: McGraw-Hill.

The quote at the beginning of the chapter and the one that follows, both from authoritative voices, suggest that getting your protein needs is quite simple.

> A dietary protein intake that represents about 15% of the total energy intake with an energy-sufficient diet should cover the requirements for nearly all endurance athletes. Given the increase in energy intake by most athletes, there is no need to use protein supplements to attain these levels.
>
> *Professor Mark Tarnopolsky,*
> Clinical Sports Nutrition, 2000

These opinions reflect the research since 1990. Most active people will use at least 10,500 kilojoules (2,500 cal) per day, and 15 per cent of that is 1,570 kilojoules (375 cal), which is around 94 grams of protein. This will cover the protein needs of many athletes, as shown in table 2.2. Although athletes need more protein than the unfit, their extra protein needs are covered by their bigger appetites, making protein a perceived, rather than a real, concern for athletes.

Dr. Peter Lemon of the University of Western Ontario, Canada, is acknowledged as one of the foremost researchers in the area of protein needs of athletes. He believes that strength or speed athletes should consume about 1.6 to 1.7 grams of protein per kilogram of body weight and that endurance athletes should consume about 1.2 to 1.4 grams of protein per kilogram of body weight. Athletes just beginning a training program might need the higher end of the range, whereas seasoned athletes probably require less protein. He doesn't believe there is any benefit in taking more than 2.0 grams of protein per kilogram of body weight, providing the athlete is consuming enough carbohydrate.

To put this in perspective, the average sedentary person eats 1.0 to 1.5 grams of protein per kilogram of body weight, the average female athlete eats 1.0 to 2.8 grams per kilogram, and the average male athlete eats 1.5 to 4.0 grams per kilogram, so there is a good chance you are getting enough protein. But don't take my word for it. Use the Nutrient Food Value Chart at the end of this book to see whether you're getting enough protein to cover your training needs.

Can You Eat Too Much Protein?

Almost everyone in Western society eats more protein than necessary. The average athlete often eats twice the recommended protein needs. If more protein is eaten than is required, the excess protein is used as muscle fuel during exercise or possibly stored as body fat (but not muscle). There is probably no harm in a healthy adult having a relatively high protein intake. Although the general view is that no athlete needs more than 2 grams of protein per kilogram of body weight, there is no evidence of harm when consuming 2.5 to 3.0 grams per kilogram (about 240 g in an 80 kg, or 176 lb, athlete).

One consideration is that protein is high in nitrogen, and this nitrogen needs to be excreted daily via the kidneys. Therefore, more protein means more urine production, which in turn requires the athlete to drink more water. Anyone with kidney or liver disease will need to see a specialist for specific protein recommendations.

The sample menu in table 2.3 provides around 127 grams of protein and 11,370 kilojoules (2,720 cal), showing that getting plenty of protein in a day is quite easy. A daily intake of 11,370 kilojoules is modest—most active people will eat more than this.

Should You Consume Protein Just Before Sport?

There is some evidence that having a small amount of protein in the form of amino acids with a carbohydrate drink improves muscle protein balance. Whether this translates to increased muscle mass or muscle strength is not clear. We are really in the early days of research regarding protein taken just prior to sport.

Should You Consume Protein During Sport?

If protein is consumed in a beverage during sport, will it reduce protein breakdown or reduce muscle damage? Although we are not certain of the answer, some early research hints that a little protein in a sports drink could be beneficial in endurance sport. Long-distance cyclists were given either a sports drink or a sports drink with added whey protein (1.8 grams per 100 mL). The cyclists who were given

Table 2.3 Sample High-Carbohydrate–High-Protein Meal Plan

Food	Protein	Fat	Carbohydrate
Weetbix, 3	6	1	30
Milk, reduced fat, 200 mL (7 oz)	8	4	12
Bread, 2 slices	5	2	30
Margarine, 2 tsp	0	8	0
Marmalade, jam, 4 tsp	0	0	14
Fruit juice, 150 mL (5 oz)	0	0	15
Banana	2	0	22
Ham and salad sandwich, 2	24	21	60
Flavoured milk, 300 mL (10 oz)	12	6	25
Flavoured yogurt, 200 mL (7 oz)	9	4	25
Sports drink, 500 mL (17 oz)	0	0	30
Steamed rice, 2 cups	10	2	100
Chicken breast, 150 g (5.3 oz)	42	6	0
Vegetables, 1 cup	3	0	10
Fruit salad, 1 cup	1	0	24
Ice cream, 1 scoop	2	5	10
Milo (2 tsp Milo + 40 mL, or 1.4 oz, milk + water)	3	2	8
Totals	127	61	415

sports drinks with added protein were able to ride for 29 per cent longer to exhaustion. The researchers also found less muscle damage in the cyclists who were given the sports drink with protein (Saunders, Kane and Todd 2004). More research is needed in this area to clarify whether protein taken during sport will help some athletes. (For more information on sports drinks, see chapter 5.)

The following questions need to be answered before we can give more precise information on protein requirements during sport: If protein during sport does increase endurance, how much protein is ideal? What is the best type of protein? Should the protein be taken in solid or liquid form?

Should You Consume Protein Straight After Sport?

It is commonly claimed that you should consume 30 grams of protein soon after a workout to promote protein uptake into the muscles. Having now interviewed three prominent researchers on protein needs (Mark Tarnopolsky, Kevin Tipton and Peter Lemon), I discovered that none of them know where this idea came from. In fact, it doesn't make logical sense. If there was a specific protein recommendation after a workout, it would be based on gender, body weight and the intensity of the workout. Yes, some protein is needed after exercise to build muscle and help repair any muscle damage, but we still don't know exactly how much protein, what type of protein would be best or when it should be eaten. The best advice we can give is to make sure you eat protein-containing foods soon after a workout and get enough protein through the day.

A regular meal including lean protein sources and high-carbohydrate foods does stimulate the uptake of amino acids, mainly through the action of the hormone insulin released after a meal. Any reasonable meal will provide around 30 grams of protein and 100 grams of carbohydrate (e.g., one ham and salad roll + one fruit + 250 mL juice is around 30 grams of protein and 85 grams of carbohydrate; a Triple G described in chapter 11 and two pieces of fruit will provide 26 grams of protein and 80 grams of carbohydrate). This should allow the body to quickly repair any muscle damage caused by a workout and provide amino acids to help increase muscle mass in strength training.

Protein Supplements

The protein supplement was born mainly in response to the demands of bodybuilders. Although protein is a popular supplement, few athletes or bodybuilders need extra protein in addition to the protein they get from food. One athlete, when shown how much protein he was getting from food, thanked me for saving him $40 a week on protein powders. That's an extra $2,080 tax-free each year in his pocket.

Some athletes can benefit from a protein supplement as they may not get enough in their diets. Vegans and other strict vegetarians may prefer to meet their extra protein needs through a soy protein supplement. Some athletes expend so much energy each day that the protein supplement becomes a simple way of getting more nutrients and calories to meet their needs.

Whether you are buying a supplement drink or meal replacement for weight loss, muscle gain or improved performance, what appear on the label are usually the scientific terms for each ingredient. That can make it sound more impressive than it is or just plain confuse you. Here are some examples:

- Calcium caseinate—milk protein
- Whey protein—another milk protein (left over from cheese manufacturing)
- Lactalbumin—milk protein
- Nonfat milk solids—nonfat milk powder
- Soy protein isolate—protein extracted from soybeans
- Egg albumin—egg white
- Dextrose—glucose
- Maltodextrins—small chains of glucose molecules
- Xantham, carrageenan, guar—vegetable gums often used as a thickening agent
- Lecithin—an emulsifier that stops any fat from rising to the top of the drink

All of the previous ingredients are inexpensive and do not generally deserve to be sold to consumers at premium prices. Even the vitamins added to such products are inexpensive.

Using the scientific name for common ingredients gives the product an almost 'magic' aura

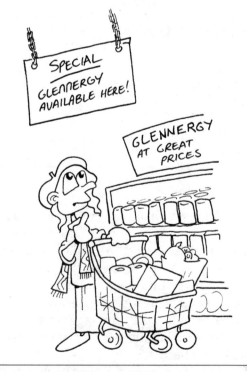

If you buy the right ingredients, you can make your own nutritional supplements.

and makes it impossible for the public to interpret the ingredient list. In a survey I conducted, protein supplements ranged from $16 to $47 per kilogram (or $7 to $21 per lb). More recently, some have topped the $80 per kilogram mark. I have a homemade protein/energy supplement that a client named after me (Glennergy DIY) that is inexpensive ($8 per kilogram) and can be made in the comfort of your own kitchen. See page 28 for the Glennergy DIY recipe. You could also try the drink recipes near the end of chapter 11. Most of them are good sources of protein.

Many protein supplements list their amino acid content. Compare them with the amino acid profile of the common foods listed in table 2.4. Fill in the blank column with information on the amino acid content of your favourite supplement. It may be cheaper to get your protein from food. Some specific amino acids are promoted as sports supplements, but there is little scientific evidence to suggest they are useful to athletes, as explained in more detail in chapter 8.

Protein powders and weight gain powders have virtually the same ingredients as weight loss powders: milk powder, soy protein, sugar, vitamins and flavour.

Table 2.4 Approximate Amino Acid Content (in Milligrams) of Some Foods

Amino acid	Protein or amino acid supplement	Baked beans, 1 cup	Milk, 250 mL (8 oz) glass	Egg, 50 g (1.8 oz)	Skim milk powder, 100 g (3.5 oz)
Isoleucine		565	495	343	2,124
Leucine		1,012	802	534	3,438
Lysine		745	650	452	2,784
Methionine		117	205	196	880
Phenylalanine		667	395	334	1,694
Threonine		373	370	302	1,584
Tryptophan		128	115	76	495
Valine		650	550	384	2,349
Histidine		330	223	149	952
Arginine		572	298	377	1,271
Alanine		507	283	350	1,210
Aspartate		1,577	622	632	2,663
Cystine		92	75	146	325
Glutamate		2,000	1,718	822	7,350
Glycine		465	173	212	743
Proline		600	795	250	3,400
Serine		800	445	468	1,909
Tyrosine		302	395	256	1,694

(continued)

Table 2.4 *(continued)*

Amino acid	Protein or amino acid supplement	Lean chicken breast, 100 g (3.5 oz)	Lean beef, 100 g (3.5 oz)	Bread, 1 slice (30 g; 1 oz)	Rice, 1 cup cooked (150 g; 5.3 oz)
Isoleucine		1638	1,198	105	153
Leucine		2,328	2,095	188	292
Lysine		2,635	2,226	85	127
Methionine		859	686	43	84
Phenylalanine		1,231	1,040	130	189
Threonine		1,310	1,052	83	126
Tryptophan		362	173	39	40
Valine		1,539	1,307	124	216
Histidine		963	840	63	84
Arginine		1,871	1,703	126	295
Alanine		1,692	1,601	75	205
Aspartate		2,764	2,399	108	333
Cystine		397	340	60	72
Glutamate		4,645	3,954	825	690
Glycine		1,524	1,604	80	162
Proline		1,275	1,255	315	166
Serine		1,067	1,037	140	186
Tyrosine		1,047	839	81	118

Data from USDA National Nutrient Database for Standard Reference, Release 17 (2004)
www.nal.usda.gov/fnic/foodcomp/Data/SR17/reports/sr17page.htm.

Glennergy DIY

If you really believe you need a protein supplement, here's one that will save you a lot of money. You can make it for around 20 per cent of the retail cost of a similar protein powder.

Bulk recipe

1 kg (2.2 lb) nonfat milk powder

7 Tbsp sugar

7 Tbsp flavour (e.g., Milo, Nesquik)

Method: Mix together to make powder. To make one drink add 4 Tbsp powder to 200 mL water.

Compare the nutrition analysis of Glennergy DIY with the nutrition label on your protein powder. Remember the following:

- Your body cannot tell the difference between protein in a protein powder and protein from milk powder. If you truly believe you need extra protein, then an affordable drink such as Glennergy is the way to go.

Nutrition Analysis

	per drink (4 Tbsp or 32 g)	per 100 g of powder	per 25 g (1/3 cup)
Protein (g)	9	27	7
Carbohydrate (g)	21	62	16
Fat (g)	<1	2	0.5
Calcium (mg)	325	980	245
Energy	510 kJ (122 cal)	1,540 kJ (370 cal)	385 kJ (93 cal)

- Your protein powder may have more protein per 100 grams than Glennergy, mainly because the carbohydrate has been extracted. Compare the cost per gram of protein.

- Glennergy also makes an ideal presport meal. You may want to blend in some fruit rather than adding flavouring.

FINAL SCORE

- Active people and athletes need more protein than spectators do.

- The current evidence doesn't suggest that performance can be significantly enhanced by protein or amino acid supplementation, except in the unlikely event that the athlete is getting inadequate protein.

- The protein needs of an athlete can be met adequately with a variety of healthy foods. Use the Nutrient Food Value Chart at the end of the manual to assess your own protein intake.

- An inexpensive milk-based protein drink such as Glennergy or Triple G (described in chapter 11) can be a useful adjunct to a healthy training diet.

- Protein can be converted to glucose to be used as a muscle fuel, but this usually occurs only near the end of endurance sports such as triathlons, marathons or ironman events, or if an excessive amount of protein is consumed.

- Future research may show that taking protein or amino acids before or during endurance exercise may reduce muscle protein breakdown to glucose.

three

Carbohydrate for Energy

Our knowledge of sports nutrition has come a long way since Robert Barclay Allardice walked 1,600 kilometres (1,000 miles) in 1,000 hours, about 38 kilometres (24 miles) a day for 42 days. In 1999 long-distance runner Pat Farmer was able to run 70 kilometres (43 miles) a day for 200 days to run around Australia by being on the right fuel. All sports scientists agree that an athlete's diet must be high in carbohydrate to fuel muscles.

Why Carbohydrate?

Carbohydrate is your main source of glucose, the sugar used by the body to produce ATP for muscle contraction (see chapter 1). If you do not stock up on carbohydrate, then your glycogen stores will be low and you will quickly run out of glycogen during exercise. Once you run out of glycogen (i.e., 'hit the wall'), you will need to rely heavily on muscle protein and body fat for energy. Unfortunately, these are less efficient than carbohydrate as fuel.

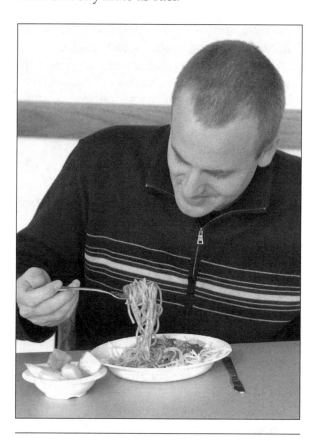

High-carbohydrate foods fuel the muscles before sport and refuel them after sport.

You may have been told to avoid carbohydrate in an attempt to lose excess body fat. This is misguided because in doing so you are depriving the body of its favourite fuel for exercise. If you are involved in aerobic exercise, then you will need carbohydrate and fat for fuel. As the intensity of exercise increases, your muscles will need mainly glucose (carbohydrate). If you do mainly weight training, then you will rely heavily on carbohydrate for fuel as each muscle contraction will use glucose. Some weight training athletes avoid carbohydrate foods not realising that their glucose is being produced from the protein they eat. That's not necessarily a problem; it's just that high-protein foods are usually more expensive than high-carbohydrate foods.

Blood Glucose and Glycogen

When you eat carbohydrate, your blood glucose level rises, which stimulates the release of the hormone insulin. Blood glucose is commonly called blood sugar, and insulin is needed to lower the blood sugar level after a meal and promote storage of glucose as muscle and liver glycogen. Some people believe that this release of insulin inevitably results in low blood sugar and, therefore, decreased sports performance. But this is misguided because in most cases the insulin brings blood glucose back to normal. Should blood glucose drop too low, another hormone called glucagon steps in to raise it back to normal. This happens in most healthy adults.

Another common misconception is that insulin converts carbohydrate to fat. This is not true. Instead, insulin promotes the storage of glucose as muscle and liver glycogen, not as fat! Insulin also helps the muscles take up amino acids for muscle repair, and fat for fuel during aerobic exercise. So, in summary, the digestive enzymes break down the starch molecules, and the resulting glucose molecules are absorbed into the bloodstream, causing a rise in the blood glucose levels. The hormone insulin then lowers the blood glucose levels and promotes storage of glucose as muscle and liver glycogen.

Athletes generally eat lots of high-carbohydrate foods, so they are able to store more glycogen, allowing them to train and compete for long periods. Glycogen is a long sequence of glucose molecules with many branches, similar to amylopectin in starch. This branching is very useful as it allows glycogen to be quickly broken down to individual glucose molecules for muscle energy during exercise.

How Much Carbohydrate Should You Eat?

Plenty, if you are a very active person. Almost all surveys of athletes reveal that they eat too little carbohydrate for their training level. Most adults eat only 150 to 250 grams of carbohydrate a day. That might be OK if you are sedentary. Unfortunately, that amount of carbohydrate daily is not enough to fuel an athlete's body, so it's no wonder so many feel tired. Most recreational athletes need 300 to 400 grams of carbohydrate daily. Elite athletes need 500 to 700 grams every day.

Just how much carbohydrate you need to eat depends on your sport, training level, gender, size, appetite and so on. I'll try to help you to find your carbohydrate needs, which will be expressed in grams of carbohydrate for every kilogram of your ideal weight (see table 3.1).

Based on table 3.1 and your body weight, you can get an approximate idea of your carbohydrate needs by using this simple formula:

Your weight (in kg) × grams
of carbohydrate per kg of body weight
= your carbohydrate needs each day

For example, from table 3.1 we can see that a serious amateur athlete might need 6 grams of carbohydrate per kilogram of body weight per day. If the athlete weighs 70 kilograms (154 lb), the equation would look like this:

70 kg × 6 g carbohydrate per kg
= 420 g carbohydrate per day

Be warned: When you do your calculations, you will see that you need a lot of carbohydrate, and you're going to think, How will I ever eat that much? If your carbohydrate needs are high, then you will likely need to eat frequent snacks or meals throughout the day just to get enough food. I'll show you later in this chapter how it's done in food terms. Make your first goal to eat a little more carbohydrate (say, an

Table 3.1   Your Carbohydrate Needs

Carbohydrate (g per kg of body weight per day)	Activity level sustained
1	The amount of carbohydrate you get with some weight loss programs Very little aerobic activity possible
2	Sleeping, watching TV, sitting
3 (The amount most adults eat)	Daily chores
4–5	A good intake for active people Walking, moderate exercise, recreational sports, fitness programs (3–5 hr/wk)
5–7	Serious amateur sports, football, rugby, netball, bodybuilding, weight training Medium level of exercise (6–10 hr/wk)
7–9	Serious professional sports Endurance sports, marathons Training 10+ hours a week
10+	Full-time athletes Ultra-endurance, Ironman events Olympic athlete Training 15+ hours a week

Note: This is a guide only. Women generally can sustain activity at the lower end of the range of carbohydrate intake for each activity level.

extra 50 grams a day). One trick is to cut back on the fatty foods to make more room for high-carbohydrate foods. You will certainly feel and perform better if you do. Less fat in your meals may take a little getting used to. Remember, it's less fat, not zero fat.

Certainly, men find it easier than women to eat enough carbohydrate. Part of this might be that women are better fat burners than men are and need less carbohydrate. They should choose the lower-carbohydrate figure for their activity level in table 3.1.

Carbohydrate Loading

The classic carbohydrate-loading regimen was first described in 1967 by Scandinavian researchers (Bergström and Hultman 1967). To boost muscle glycogen stores, their athletes endured three days of low-carbohydrate eating, followed by three days of high-carbohydrate eating just before the big event. This regimen does increase the amount of glycogen stored in muscle, but in the three days without carbohydrate the athlete suffers severe fatigue and irritability and feels like an invalid with a sack of potatoes under each arm. This manner of increasing glycogen stores is no longer considered necessary, although some athletes still swear by it.

Now we realise that a high-carbohydrate diet throughout the pre-event week, especially the two days before, has the same effect of raising muscle glycogen to high levels as the Scandinavian regimen. For this reason sports dietitians recommend high-carbohydrate eating all the time for serious athletes. Enjoyable carbohydrate loading now consists of a week of tapered training, working down to light training in the three days before the event, while at the same time consuming high-carbohydrate meals. This

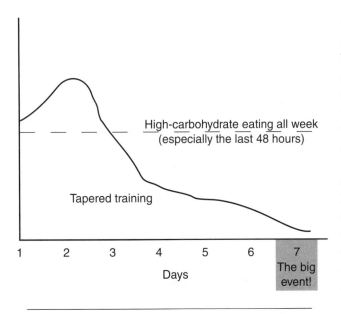

Figure 3.1 Carbohydrate loading combined with tapered training in the week before a big endurance event.

pattern is illustrated in figure 3.1. Be aware that as training tapers, you are likely to feel less hungry than you usually do. Just make sure that the foods you choose are relatively high in carbohydrate.

This message can get confused. Some see carbohydrate loading as cake overloading. Carbohydrate loading is not an excuse to eat until you are bloated! The idea is to eat plenty of carbohydrate, not lots of any food that tastes sweet. Cake may taste sweet, but a lot of its kilojoules (40 per cent) comes from fat.

Pasta is a favourite pre-event meal for most athletes. Unfortunately, many think that just because they have pasta on their plate, they're carbohydrate loading. It's not the case, however, if the pasta is suffocating under a mountain of meat sauce and cheese. Pasta should be the mountain; and the sauce and cheese, the snow cap.

An athlete might eat more bread for extra carbohydrate, yet be totally unaware that a 290 kilojoule (70 cal) slice of bread has been smeared with 420 kilojoules (100 cal) or more of margarine or butter. This is 'fat loading', not carbohydrate loading. It's smarter to have only a scrape of butter or margarine to allow enough room for two slices of bread. Likewise, potato should not be served with lots of sour cream, and rice shouldn't be fried with lots of oil. In both cases more energy is coming from fat than from carbohydrate.

Sugar and Your Health

You will note that some of my suggestions to boost carbohydrate include foods that have sugar such as sorbet, confectionery (candy) and ice cream. Fortunately, active people have a great deal of flexibility with their diet and can include some sugar-containing food without compromising their health. Some foods with sugar such as flavoured yogurt, ice cream and chocolate also provide essential nutrients.

Boosting the Carbohydrate (But Not the Fat)

- Eat at least two pieces of fruit a day.
- Eat plenty of starchy vegetables, such as peas, corn, potato, baked beans.
- If you like hot chips or french fries, choose low-fat oven fries (frozen food section).
- Eat all kinds of pasta (go easy on cheese and oil).
- Choose low-fat milk and yogurt (flavoured versions OK).
- Eat steamed rice instead of fried rice.
- Eat fruit instead of biscuits, cookies or cakes.
- Eat a bread roll instead of pies, pastries or sausage rolls.
- Breakfast cereals are high in carbohydrate (avoid toasted varieties).
- Eat more bread, but use less butter or margarine.
- Try a banana sandwich for a carbohydrate-packed snack.
- Halve the oil, margarine or butter in standard recipes—doing so usually doesn't affect the end result and makes more room for carbohydrate.
- Have lots of canned fruit and one scoop of ice cream for dessert.
- Sorbet and gelato make great desserts.

Sugar confectionery is used by many athletes as a carbohydrate source during, or just after, sport. Let's take a brief look at two issues that usually arise when sugar is discussed.

Sugar in Food

Part of the emotion of the debate of sugar versus starch is that most people don't understand the real difference between the two. It is not rational to state that sugar-containing foods are implicitly 'bad' given that foods such as fruit, milk, yogurt and soy drinks provide their carbohydrate only as sugars (e.g., fruit provides glucose, fructose and sucrose; milk provides lactose). Some of the sweeter vegetables also contain sugar. Because fruits provide a handsome dividend in antioxidants (chemicals that slow the aging of the body), it would be ridiculous to malign them based on their sugar content.

The real problem is not sugar per se but 'added sugar' (sugar not naturally present in a food). Added-sugar foods can displace more nutritious foods from the diet. A can of soft drink will easily fit into an active person's diet, but 2 litres a day is not wise nutrition for anyone.

There is no scientific link between sugar and diabetes, heart disease, arthritis or any other disease you care to name. The reason many adults get adult-onset diabetes is that their bodies have a reduced sensitivity to insulin and their blood sugar levels rise to unhealthy levels. This is commonly due to being over-weight, itself caused by overeating and under-exercising. Remember that table sugar is merely fructose and glucose, two molecules we have been consuming for millennia. Although sugar does not cause life-threatening disease, it may be involved in dental disease.

Sugar and Your Teeth

If you don't take care of your teeth, excess sugar in your diet could cause tooth decay. Any carbohydrate (both sugar and starch) that remains in the mouth after meals can be converted to lactic acid by bacteria in the mouth. The lactic acid can then eat away at the enamel of the tooth and, over time, cause decay. It is not scientific, however, to blame solely sugar for tooth decay. All forms of carbohydrate, including dried fruit and bread, have the potential to cause tooth decay.

There are a number of ways to stop tooth decay. Naturally, saliva has tooth-protective elements, and regular brushing and flossing of teeth also help maintain dental hygiene. Saliva also helps raise the pH to buffer the acids produced by bacteria or taken in the diet. For example, sports drinks, soft drinks and fruit juices are quite acidic and shouldn't stay in the mouth in contact with teeth for too long.

Looking after your teeth is more a case of dental hygiene than of avoiding sugar. Dentists recommend that you have at least two hours between eating times to allow time for saliva to raise the pH and repair any damage caused to tooth enamel.

Guinness Book of Records

Although I do recommend that you eat an adequate amount of carbohydrate and enjoy your meals, some people have taken carbohydrate eating to the extreme. Years ago, the Guinness Book of Records documented individual cases of gluttony before they stopped those kinds of records. The 27th edition of the GBR contained a few records for eating carbohydrate foods (McWhirter 1980). How's this for carbohydrate loading?

- Martin Moore ate 2,380 baked beans one by one with a cocktail stick in half an hour.

- Dr. Ronald Alkana ate 17 bananas (2.2 kg [4.8 lb]) in two minutes way back in 1973.

- It took only 82 seconds for Peter Dowdeswell of England to chug down 1.4 kilograms (3 lb) of potatoes. Peter also has an earlier record for eating 40 jam butties (jam sandwiches) in just under 18 minutes.

- Finally, 91.5 metres (300 ft) of spaghetti slid down the throat of Steve Weldon in 29 seconds. Wel-don, Steve!

Smart Carbohydrate Eating

The idea of getting 400 grams of carbohydrate or more each day may sound like a lot of eating. Well, it isn't, if you choose wisely. Following are three sample menus that provide over 400 grams of carbohydrate.

High-Carbohydrate Menu 1

Food, Carbohydrate (g)			
Breakfast		**Snack**	
4 Weetbix, Vita Brits	40	1 apple	14
200 mL reduced-fat milk (7 oz)	12	300 mL flavoured milk (10 oz)	25
2 tsp sugar	10	**Training**	
2 slices toast	30	1,000 mL sports drink	60
1 Tbsp jam/marmalade	14	**Dinner**	
Snack		Meat	0
1 bread muffin	28	2 medium potatoes	32
1 banana	22	1 cup peas	9
Lunch		1 cup carrots	5
4 slices bread + lean meat + salad (sandwich)	60	2 scoops ice cream	20
		1 cup canned fruit	21
250 mL fruit juice (8 oz)	25	250 mL fruit juice (8 oz)	25
1 chocolate bar, 50 g (1.8 oz)	30		
		Total carbohydrate	**482**

High-Carbohydrate Menu 2

Food, Carbohydrate (g)			
Breakfast		**Snack**	
1 cup canned spaghetti	30	1 flavoured milk, 300 mL (10 oz)	25
4 slices toast	60	**Dinner**	
250 mL fruit juice (8 oz)	25	2 cups steamed rice	100
Snack		Meat/chicken/fish	0
Food bar	25	Stir-fried vegetables	15
Lunch		1 cup fruit salad	24
2 bread rolls + avocado + salad	60	Yogurt, flavoured nonfat	25
1 banana	22		
1 iced fruit bun	40		
		Total carbohydrate	**451**

High-Carbohydrate Menu 3

Food, Carbohydrate (g)			
Breakfast		**Snack**	
2 cups breakfast cereal	50	2 mandarins	12
200 mL reduced-fat milk (7 oz)	12	**Dinner**	
2 tsp sugar	10	1 cup meat or seafood sauce	0
1/2 cup canned fruit	11	2 cups pasta	100
Snack		Side salad	5
1 breakfast bar	28	2 scoops ice cream	20
1 medium apple	14	1 cup canned fruit	21
Lunch		250 mL fruit juice (8 oz)	25
2 bread rolls + chicken + salad	60		
Triple G (see chapter 11)	47		
		Total carbohydrate	**415**

Carbohydrate Confusion

Following are two examples of an athlete who has eaten enough calories but hasn't reached his carbohydrate goals. As a result, he faded badly during training. This person thought he was getting enough carbohydrate because he ate carbohydrate foods at each meal. Unfortunately, his choices were not ideal (e.g., french fries provide 40 per cent of their energy as fat), or they were inadequate (one cup of pasta is not likely to be enough for an active person).

Carbohydrate Fadeout 1

Food, Carbohydrate (g)

Breakfast		Snack	
2 slices toast + margarine	30	Doughnut	20
1 cup white tea	2	**Dinner**	
1 tsp sugar	5	1 cup pasta	50
Lunch		Meat sauce	0
Bacon and cheese hamburger	50	Parmesan cheese	0
French fries	50		
375 mL diet soft drink (13 oz)	0		
		Total carbohydrate	**207**

Carbohydrate Fadeout 2

Food, Carbohydrate (g)

Breakfast		Snack	
2 slices toast	30	Flavoured milk, 300 mL (10 oz)	25
2 eggs	0	**Dinner**	
2 rashers bacon	0	3 pieces fried chicken	0
200 mL fruit juice (7 oz)	20	1 cup mashed potato	30
Snack		Vegetables	10
2 biscuits	14		
Lunch			
1 bread roll with filling	30		
1 slice of cake	36		
		Total carbohydrate	**195**

Meeting Your Carbohydrate Needs

Although your regular meals will provide the majority of your carbohydrate needs, sometimes other products can help supplement your carbohydrate intake. We will take a look at three of these.

Food Bars

There is a great range of food bars to choose from. Some are marketed as sports bars and energy bars, but these are nowhere near as magical as they might imply. Although they are generally a good-quality product and low in fat, you can usually get better value for your money with a wisely chosen muesli bar, fruit bar or breakfast bar. Many specialty food bars claim to encourage body fat loss or increase your endurance or strength. They are unlikely to have a singular benefit based solely on the protein, fat, carbohydrate and added nutrients. I know there is a wonderful attraction to bars promising you the result you seek, but they are probably no substitute for good, wholesome eating and hard training. Beware of food bars claiming to 'mobilise' body fat or increase the amount of fat used as muscle fuel. There is no evidence to support their claims.

Use the 4 and 20 rule of food bars: As a general rule, any food bar providing less than 4 grams of fat and more than 20 grams of carbohydrate is a good choice. See the snack section in the Nutrient Food Value Chart at the end of the book for some examples. Food bars are convenient for pre- and postevent snacks as they don't need refrigeration and can be sat upon and don't spoil so they can be stashed in a gym bag for days. Remember, bars are not a substitute for meals, just a quick and handy snack to have in your sports bag or car to tide you over to your next meal.

Carbohydrate Supplements

During high-level training, many athletes have difficulty eating enough food to match the calorie and carbohydrate needs of their bodies. This is particularly common in elite athletes and endurance athletes training many hours a day. They have less rest time for eating and don't want too much food in their stomachs when exercising. If this sounds like you, then you may benefit from carbohydrate supplements and liquid meal supplements.

Some carbohydrate supplements are available in the form of gels or powdered sugars. Generally these are glucose based (e.g., Glucodin, Carboshotz) as glucose is one of the least sweet sugars and can be added to fruit juices, drinks and canned fruit. Like sports bars, carbohydrate supplements are convenient and easy to carry, but they aren't magic. It may be cheaper to get your extra carbohydrate as fruit juice, food bars, breakfast cereals, sports drinks, cordials or soft drinks (soda).

Because liquids are generally easier to consume than solids, liquid meals and snacks can be very helpful in meeting athletes' high-energy needs. Commercial varieties are available, or you can make your own (see chapter 11, p. 147).

Snacks

Snacking is another way to meet your carbohydrate needs. When you are so hungry that food dominates your thoughts, think smart and snack smart. Sure, a piece of fruit is still the quickest nutritious snack around, but sometimes it doesn't fill the spot, nor is it convenient. Food bars are a favourite with athletes—fruit bars, breakfast bars, muesli bars, sports bars or even chocolate bars.

Snacks of all types can offer good nutrition—fruit muffins, toast, fruit bread, half a sandwich or roll, cracker breads, yogurt, baked potato, dried fruit, flavoured milk, doner kebab, popcorn or baked beans. Even cereal and milk is a quick snack any time of the day. A low-fat treat could include sorbet, confectionery, soft drinks or fruit juice. Your imagination will provide more ideas.

The more active you are, the more likely you are to need a snack and the more freedom you have with your food choices. For example, a soft drink may provide only sugar and water, but if it is only a small part of a 12,000+ kilojoule (3,000+ cal) diet, there's still plenty of room for more nutritious food choices. You are smart enough to get the balance right. It's not whether you snack, it's what you snack on that will affect your performance and your health.

Glycemic Index

Back in the old days we used to divide carbohydrate into 'simple' and 'complex' forms. It was generally agreed that simple forms of carbohydrate were honey, syrups, soft drinks, confectionery and sugars (glucose, fructose, sucrose, maltose, dextrose); and complex forms were breads, rice, pasta, cereals, fruits and starchy vegetables. It was assumed that all simple forms of carbohydrate were digested quickly and complex forms were digested slowly. As scientists discover more amazing things about food, nature and human beings, it should be no surprise that our understanding becomes more refined. And so it is with carbohydrate.

Some of the 'simple' forms of carbohydrate aren't so simple, and some of the 'complex' forms aren't as complex as we thought. Now a carbohydrate food can be classified by how quickly it is digested and absorbed into the blood as glucose; this classification is known as its glycemic index (GI). The GI is essentially the measurement of the blood glucose response to eating foods with carbohydrate. There is no GI for a food without carbohydrate such as meat or oil.

Determining GI

The GI of a food is determined from eating the amount of that food that provides 50 grams of carbohydrate, and then measuring its effect on blood glucose levels (see figure 3.2). For

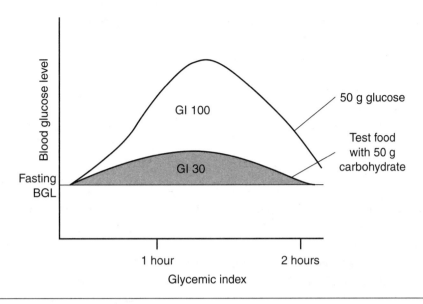

Figure 3.2 The blood glucose response to 50 grams of glucose is given a GI of 100. The blood glucose response to other foods with carbohydrate are compared to glucose.

example, three large apples will provide a total of 50 grams of carbohydrate. All foods have been compared to 50 grams of glucose, which has been given an arbitrary figure of 100. A GI of 70 means that a food with 50 grams of carbohydrate raises blood glucose levels around 70 per cent of 50 grams of pure glucose.

The basis of the glycemic index is the rate of digestion of all carbohydrates. High GI foods are quickly converted to blood glucose, and low GI foods are slowly converted to blood glucose. Some of the results of testing for GI have been surprising: Sugar has a lower GI than bread and potato! That finding has resulted in relaxing the restrictions on people with diabetes; they can now include some sugar in their diets.

'Slow' Starch and 'Quick' Starch

Starch comes in two main forms, amylose and amylopectin. All starchy foods are a mixture of the two forms of starch (see figure 3.3).

- Amylose is a straight chain of glucose molecules and takes longer to digest.
- Amylopectin has a number of branches of smaller glucose chains and is quicker to digest.

The enzyme that breaks down starch can work only on the end glucose molecules, breaking them off in chunks of one or two molecules. Amylose, being a straight chain of

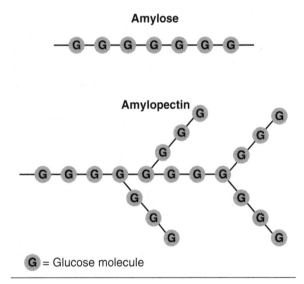

Figure 3.3 Amylopectin starch is composed of branched chains of glucose molecules; amylose is a straight chain of glucose molecules.

glucose molecules, has two end molecules. It will take longer to digest than amylopectin, which has a number of branches of glucose chains, and therefore many end molecules. For this reason starchy foods will have different rates of digestion. Starches high in amylopectin will digest more quickly and have a greater effect on blood glucose than will starches high in amylose. For example, bread is made from wheat, which is high in amylopectin. Pasta, on the other hand, is made from durum wheat, which is high in amylose. Therefore, bread will have a higher GI than pasta because it is digested more quickly.

Note that the GI of maltose, glucose and honey are high because of their high glucose content, whereas another sugar, fructose, has a low GI because it has little effect on blood sugar levels. Table sugar (sucrose) is a molecule made of glucose and fructose joined together; hence, its GI is halfway between glucose and fructose (68 in table 3.2 on page 42). The least processed starchy foods are generally slower to digest and have a lower GI. This can be very relevant to people with diabetes because the lower the rise in blood glucose levels, the easier it is to control diabetes. The processing of starchy foods can break the amylose into smaller pieces, providing more end glucose molecules and enabling quicker digestion. Later, I will mention other factors that influence the GI of a food.

GI and Nutritional Value

If you are thinking that the GI of a food is some kind of league table of nutritional value and that those with the least GI are better for you than those with the highest GI, then hold up a moment. First, be aware that a food does not have a set GI, but a range of GIs. The GI for rice can be as low as 56 (e.g., Doongara rice, which is higher in amylose) or as high as 90 for those that are low in amylose. The variation is due to the different botanical types having different proportions of the two types of starch. Under-ripe bananas will have a GI of 40, whereas ripe bananas will be around 50 or 60 because the ripening process produces a higher level of glucose. So don't get hung up on the absolute GI number. The GI allows you to compare different foods within the same food grouping, such as breakfast cereals.

Second, remember that the GI is a comparison of carbohydrate foods based on 50 grams of carbohydrate. Some foods you generally won't eat in amounts that provide 50 grams of carbohydrate; for example, most serves of fruit will provide only 15 grams of carbohydrate and a medium boiled potato has 25 grams of carbohydrate. Although it is uncommon for a serve of food to provide 50 grams of carbohydrate, a cup of cooked spaghetti has pretty close to that amount.

Glycemic Load

Because we don't eat carbohydrate foods in an amount that always provides 50 grams of carbohydrate, the concept of the glycemic load (GL) was established.

$$GL = \frac{\text{Grams of carbohydrate per serve} \times GI}{100}$$

For example, the watermelon has an average GI of 72, which is classified as high, but you would eat only a 120-gram serve providing only 6 grams carbohydrate (not the 50 grams on which the GI is based). Therefore, the glycemic load (GL) is $6 \times 72 / 100 = 4.32$, or 4 to the nearest whole number. Compare that to a bagel, which also has an average GI of 72, but a single bagel provides 35 grams of carbohydrate. The GL of a bagel is $35 \times 72 / 100 = 25$. That's two foods with the same GI, but one has potentially six times the effect on blood glucose levels of the other when eaten in normal serves. The point I am trying to make is that you need not be overly concerned about the GI of foods. A high GI food such as watermelon is natural and nutritious, so you wouldn't avoid it based on its GI. For health and sport you should ask two important questions: (1) Is it minimally processed? and (2) Does it meet my carbohydrate goals?

Don't get the impression that you should check only the GL; if you do, you could end up eating very little carbohydrate and find yourself tiring very quickly in sport and exercise. Take a look at table 3.2. Although the foods have been listed in order of descending GI, the GL per serve varies greatly.

This then presents another issue. Many of the foods listed won't be eaten on their own. The bagel is likely to have a filling, which will affect the GI of the meal. The GI of a meal is approximately the average of the GI of the individual foods based on their carbohydrate content. So, if half of the carbohydrate in a meal came from rice (GI 83) and the other half from kidney beans (GI 27), then the GI of the meal would be around 55 (83 + 27 = 110; divide 110 by 2 and you get 55). Tables 3.3 and 3.4 show the GI and GL, respectively, of foods by food group.

What Can Influence GI?

Many other aspects of a meal can affect its GI and GL. Other components of the meal, such as fat, soluble fibre and protein, usually lower the GI, whereas cooking and processing usually raise the GI. Fat, fibre and protein lower the GI of the meal purely because they get in the way of the enzymes that break down the carbohydrate in the intestine. Imagine you are in a large room and you see a friend on the other side. It would take no time for you to walk over and greet your friend. Imagine now that same room full of people. It will take you longer to get over to the other side of the room to talk to your friend. Similarly, in the gut, fat molecules, fibre and chains of amino acids can get in the way of carbohydrate enzymes.

Highly processed foods generally have a high GI because processing breaks up the starch molecules into smaller chains. If, for example, you have one long amylose molecule, you have only two ends for the digestive enzymes to work on. If that chain gets broken in half, you now have four ends to digest. If they, in turn, are broken in half, there are now eight ends and potentially it could be digested four times as quickly, giving rise to a higher blood glucose level.

Use the GI to compare GI foods within the same group. Use the GL to compare different foods with varying carbohydrate content; for example, pumpkin has a high GI, but a low GL. So, just because it has a high GI doesn't mean that it will significantly raise your blood glucose levels.

GI and Your Health

The GI and the GL can be somewhat confusing. Many people believe that high GI foods are bad for their long-term health, yet the GI is not the best way to determine the benefits of a food. This is the main thing to remember: The GI hasn't really changed our nutrition advice to healthy, fit people. If you eat plenty of wholesome food that has been minimally processed, such as fruits, vegetables and whole-grain cereals, and have the occasional treat, your diet is likely to have a low GI. Scientists generally agree that low GI foods such as legumes, vegetables and whole-grain breads may help to prevent disease such as type 2 diabetes and heart disease. Low GI foods are generally more filling and better able to control your appetite such that you don't overeat and put on body fat. Low GI foods are also usually lower in kilojoules/calories than high GI foods are, another factor in helping you not to overeat. Evidence also suggests that eating lots of high GI foods puts a strain on insulin production, to the extent that it can cause insulin resistance

and type 2 diabetes. So, eat well and your future will likely be a healthy one.

Applying GI to Training and Competition

Now that we've explored the glycemic index of food in general, let's look at how athletes can use this information in training and competition. Choosing carbohydrate food and drinks based on their GI may provide a sports performance edge in some situations, especially when considering what to eat just before, during and just after exercise.

Before Exercise

You may have heard that athletes should eat low GI foods a couple of hours before exercise for a long and sustained release of glucose into the blood during exercise. This advice was based mainly on research conducted in the early 1990s. Studies in which athletes exercised until exhaustion (e.g., in long tennis matches, ultramarathons and Ironman events) often showed that low GI foods improved endurance. Because most of us don't exercise to the point of collapse, however, some scientists argue that the GI is not relevant to normal exercise, especially exercise that lasts less than 90 minutes. Research shows that the GI of the food or meal eaten before sport won't make a big difference to regular performance. The most important thing is that you eat enough carbohydrate before exercise so that you will have enough glycogen for sport. On the other hand, the GI of what you consume during and after sport could make a difference.

During Exercise

During exercise, experts recommend that athletes consume only food and drink with a high GI to access the glucose quickly. Taking carbohydrate during prolonged exercise, such as taking a sports drink, makes more glucose available to the muscles so athletes can exercise for longer. Because sugars generally have a moderate to high GI, they will be easily digested and absorbed. The only exception is fructose, which is easily absorbed but takes some time to be converted to glucose for muscle contraction; hence, it is used sparingly in sports drinks (high-fructose sports drinks are not recommended for this reason).

Sports drinks such as Gatorade have a GI of around 74 because they need to be quickly absorbed into the blood to replace the glucose burned during exercise. Avoid sports drinks that claim they have a low GI (you want the sugars now, not when you have finished exercise!). Low GI foods are not usually taken during sport, except in ultra-endurance events. In this case you will need to experiment with foods to make sure they don't cause gut discomfort. Jelly beans, with a GI of 78, are very popular blood glucose replacers in sports such as cycling, rugby, football, basketball and netball.

After Exercise

There is good evidence that moderate to high GI foods eaten after exercise are converted into muscle glycogen more readily than are low GI foods. Eating high GI foods such as rice and potato, along with sports drinks, can be especially useful if you have two or

more training sessions or events in a day or you are involved in round-robin competitions that require you to play each day. However, if you have longer than 24 hours between training sessions or events, the GI seems less important for glycogen replacement over that time. It is more important that you eat enough great-tasting foods rich in carbohydrate rather than being unduly concerned about the GI of your meals.

The GI of foods is an area of active research, so we may have to refine the advice once more studies are done. If you feel that your choice of food affects your performance based on their GI, then listen to your body and choose low to moderate GI foods before sport, and higher GI foods after sport in your recovery meal.

For more information on GI and GL, get the book called *The New Glucose Revolution* by J. Brand-Miller or visit the Web site www.glycemicindex.com.

Table 3.2 Average Glycemic Index (GI) and Glycemic Load (GL) of Carbohydrate (CHO) Foods

Food	GI per serve	CHO per serve	GL per serve
High glycemic index (>70)			
Glucodin tablets, 50 g (1.8 oz)	102	50	50
Glucose, 50 g (1.8 oz)	100	50	50
Parsnip, 80 g (2.8 oz)	97	12	12
Lucozade, 250 mL (8 oz)	95	42	40
Rice Bubbles (Kellogg's), 30 g (1 oz)	87	26	22
Potato, baked, av., 1 medium	85	30	26
Potato, instant, 150 g (5.3 oz)	85	20	17
Rice (Calrose), 1 cup, cooked	83	43	36
Rice cakes, 25 g (0.9 oz)	82	21	17
Crispbread, puffed, 25 g (0.9 oz)	81	19	15
Rice (Sunbrown quick), 1 cup	80	38	31
Puffed wheat (Sanitarium), 30 g (1 oz)	80	21	17
Morning coffee biscuits, 2	79	19	15
Jelly beans, av., 30 g (1 oz)	78	28	22
Water crackers, 25 g (0.9 oz)	78	18	14
Breakfast bar, av., 30 g (1 oz)	78	23	18
Bread, whole meal, 1 slice	77	12	9
Coco Pops (Kellogg's), 30 g (1 oz)	77	26	20

Food	GI per serve	CHO per serve	GL per serve
High glycemic index (>70)			
Cornflakes, 30 g (1 oz)	77	25	20
Waffles, 35 g (1.2 oz)	76	13	10
Lebanese bread, white	75	16	12
Shredded wheat, av., 30 g (1 oz)	75	20	15
Pumpkin, 80 g (2.8 oz)	75	4	3
Mashed potato, av., 150 g (5.3 oz)	74	20	15
Sports drink, av., 250 mL (8 oz)	74	16	13
Sultana bran (Kellogg's) 30 g (1 oz)	73	19	14
Miniwheats (filled) 30 g (1 oz)	72	20	15
Bagel, 1 white, 70 g (2.5 oz)	72	35	25
Swede, 150 g (5.3 oz)	72	10	7
Popcorn, plain, 20 g (0.7 oz)	72	11	8
Watermelon, 120 g (4.2 oz)	72	6	4
Kavli crispbreads, 25 g (0.9 oz)	71	16	12
Medium glycemic index (55–70)			
Lifesavers, 30 g (1 oz)	70	30	21
Sao biscuits, 25 g (0.9 oz)	70	17	12
Bread, white, av., 1 slice	70	14	10
Weetbix (Sanitarium), 30 g (1 oz)	69	17	12
Special K (Kellogg's USA), 30 g (1 oz)	69	21	14
Crumpets, 2	69	19	13
Bread, fibre-enriched, 1 slice	68	14	9
Fanta soft drink, 250 mL (8 oz)	68	34	23
Gnocchi, 1 cup cooked	68	48	33
Sustain (Kellogg's), 30 g (1 oz)	68	22	15
Sucrose (table sugar), 10 g (0.4 oz)	68	10	7
Weetbix Multi-Grain (Sanitarium), 30 g (1 oz)	68	20	14
Taco shells, 2 shells, 20 g (0.7 oz)	68	12	8
Croissant, 65 g (2.3 oz)	67	26	17
One minute oats, av., 250 g (9 oz)	66	26	17
Cordial, diluted, 250 mL (8 oz)	66	20	13
Pineapple, 120 g (4.2 oz)	66	10	6
Nutrigrain (Kellogg's), 30 g (1 oz)	66	15	10
Milk arrowroot biscuits, 2	65	19	12
Couscous, 150 g (5.3 oz), cooked	65	35	23
Rockmelon/cantaloupe, 120 g (4.2 oz)	65	6	4

(continued)

Table 3.2 (continued)

Food	GI per serve	CHO per serve	GL per serve
Medium glycemic index (55–70)			
Vita Brits (Uncle Tobys), 30 g (1 oz)	64	20	13
Ryvita, 25 g (0.9 oz)	64	16	11
Beetroot, canned, 80 g (2.8 oz)	64	7	5
Raisins, 30 g (1 oz)	64	22	14
Mars bar, 60 g (2 oz)	62	40	25
Sweet potato, av., 1 medium	61	28	17
Figs, dried, 30 g (1 oz)	61	13	8
Muesli bar, with dried fruit, 30 g (1 oz)	61	21	13
Ice cream, average, 1 scoop	61	13	8
Just Right cereal, 30 g (1 oz)	60	22	13
Digestive biscuit, av., 2	59	16	10
Mini Wheats, plain, 30 g (1 oz)	58	21	12
Bread, rye, av., 1 slice	58	14	8
Rice, basmati, 1 cup	58	40	22
Porridge, av., 1 cup	58	22	13
Kiwi fruit, 2 medium	58	12	7
Potato crisps, plain, 50 g (1.8 oz)	57	18	10
Bread, pita, 30 g (1 oz)	57	17	10
Muesli, Swiss, 30 g (1 oz)	56	16	9
Rice (Doongara), 1 cup	56	40	22
Power bar, av., 65 g (2.3 oz)	56	42	24
Paw paw, 120 g (4.2 oz)	56	8	5
Sultanas, 30 g (1 oz)	56	23	13
Jatz, 25 g (0.9 oz)	55	17	10
Semolina, dry, 65 g (2.3 oz)	55	50	28
Honey, av., 25 g (0.9 oz)	55	18	10
Oat bran, 10 g (0.4 oz)	55	5	3
Low glycemic index (<55)			
Bread, multigrain, 1 slice	54	15	8
Special K (Kellogg's Australia), 30 g (1 oz)	54	21	11
Buckwheat, av., 150 g (5.3 oz)	54	30	16
Coca-Cola, 250 mL (8 oz)	53	26	14
Sweet corn, av., 150 g (5.3 oz)	53	32	17
Peaches, canned, natural juice, 250 g (9 oz)	52	18	9
Banana (ripe), 1 medium	51	24	12

Food	GI per serve	CHO per serve	GL per serve
Low glycemic index (<55)			
Mango, 120 g (4.2 oz)	51	15	8
Fruit bread, av., 1 slice	51	15	8
Orange juice, 250 mL (8 oz)	50	26	13
Potato, 1 boiled, av.	50	30	15
Ice cream, low fat, 1 scoop	50	6	3
Carrots, boiled, 80 g (2.8 oz)	49	5	2
Baked beans, canned, av., 150 g (5.3 oz)	48	15	7
Peas, green, av., 1/2 cup	48	7	3
Two-minute noodles, av., 180 g (6.3 oz)	47	40	19
Grapes, av., 120 g (4.2 oz)	46	18	8
Lactose, 10 g (0.4 oz)	46	10	5
Pineapple juice, unswtnd., 250 mL (8 oz)	46	34	15
Chocolate, white, 50 g (1.8 oz)	44	29	13
Sustagen Sport, 250 mL (8 oz)	43	49	21
Custard, homemade, 100 mL (3.4 oz)	43	17	7
Muesli, toasted, 30 g (1 oz)	43	17	7
Peach, fresh, av., 1 large	42	11	5
Orange, av., 1 medium	42	11	5
Milk chocolate, 50 g (1.8 oz)	42	31	13
Spaghetti, white, boiled, 1 cup	42	47	20
Choc Nesquik + milk, 250 mL (8 oz)	41	11	5
Snickers bar, 60 g (2 oz)	41	36	15
Apple juice, av., 250 mL (8 oz)	40	28	11
Fettuccine, boiled, 1 cup	40	46	18
Ravioli, boiled, meat filled, 1 cup	39	38	15
Plums, 120 g (4.2 oz)	39	12	5
Apple, av., 1 medium	38	15	6
Pear, av., 1 medium	38	11	4
Ice cream, premium, 1 scoop	37	9	4
Yam, av., 150 g (5.3 oz)	37	36	13
Spaghetti, whole-meal, 1 cup	37	42	16
Soy drink, 250 mL (8 oz)	36	18	6
Milo in milk, 250 mL (8 oz)	36	26	9
Vermicelli, boiled, 1 cup	35	44	16
Milk, flavoured, 250 mL (8 oz)	34	26	9

(continued)

Table 3.2 *(continued)*

Food	GI per serve	CHO per serve	GL per serve
Low glycemic index (<55)			
M&Ms, peanut, 30 g (1 oz)	33	17	6
Nutella, 20 g (0.7 oz)	33	12	4
Yogurt, flavoured, low fat, 200 g (7 oz)	33	31	10
Milk, nonfat, 250 mL (8 oz)	32	13	4
Milk, full cream, 250 mL (8 oz)	31	12	4
Butter beans, cooked, 150 g (5.3 oz)	31	20	6
All-Bran (Kellogg's), 30 g (1 oz)	30	15	4
Lentils, av., cooked, 1 cup	30	17	5
Apricot, dried, 60 g (2 oz)	30	27	8
Chick peas, boiled, 150 g (5.3 oz)	28	30	8
Kidney beans, cooked, av.,150 g (5.3 oz)	28	25	7
Grapefruit, av., 120 g (4.2 oz)	25	11	3
Cherries, 120 g (4.2 oz)	22	12	3
Fructose, 10 g (0.4 oz)	19	10	2
Rice bran, 30 g (1 oz)	19	14	3
Yogurt, low fat, diet, 200 g (7 oz)	14	13	4
Peanuts, roasted, 50 g (1.8 oz)	14	6	1

av. = average.

Adapted from S.K. Foster-Powell, H.A. Holt and J.C. Brand-Miller, 2002, "International table of glycemic index and glycemic load values: 2002," *Am J Clin Nutr* 76(1): 5-56. Adapted with permission by the *American Journal of Clinical Nutrition*. © Am J Clin Nutr. American Society for Clinical Nutrition.

Table 3.3 Average Glycemic Index: Sample Foods by Food Group

Food	Low GI (<55)	Medium GI (55–70)	High GI (>70)
Breads, crisp-breads	Multigrain bread Fruit bread	Bread Pita bread Crumpet Ryvita, Jatz	Bagel Lebanese bread Crispbread Water crackers
Breakfast cereals	All Bran Toasted muesli Special K (Australia)	Sustain, Just Right Shredded wheat Special K (USA) Nutrigrain Vita Brits, Weetbix Weetbix Multi-Grain Miniwheats, plain Porridge, oat bran Swiss muesli	Sultana Bran Rice Bubbles Puffed wheat Coco Pops Cornflakes Shredded Wheat Breakfast bar Mini Wheats, flavoured
Pasta and rice	Pasta, spaghetti Ravioli Two-minute noodles Rice bran	Doongara rice Basmati rice Gnocchi	White rice Rice cakes Brown rice
Vegetables, legumes	Baked beans Legumes Carrots, peas Yam, sweet corn Boiled potato	Sweet potato Beetroot	Parsnip Potato—mashed, baked, instant Pumpkin Swede
Fruit	Dried apricot Orange, banana Grapes, cherries Apple, pear Peach, fresh and canned Grapefruit, mango Plums	Pineapple Rockmelon Raisins, sultanas Paw paw Kiwi fruit	Watermelon
Dairy foods	Milk—all types Yogurt—all types Ice cream (low fat) Ice cream (premium) Custard	Ice cream (regular)	
Snacks and confectionery	White chocolate Milk chocolate Snickers bar M&Ms Peanuts	Sweet muffins Mars bar, Lifesavers Muesli bars Potato crisps Power bar	Jelly beans Some biscuits
Sports drinks, soft drinks, fruit juice	Fruit juice Coca-Cola Sustagen Sport	Fanta	Lucozade Sports drinks
Sugars	Fructose Lactose	Sucrose Honey	Glucose Maltose Glucodin (glucose powder)

Adapted from S.K. Foster-Powell, H.A. Holt and J.C. Brand-Miller, 2002, "International table of glycemic index and glycemic load values: 2002," *Am J Clin Nutr* 76(1): 5-56. Adapted with permission by the *American Journal of Clinical Nutrition*. © Am J Clin Nutr. American Society for Clinical Nutrition.

Table 3.4 Average Glycemic Load Per Serve: Sample Foods by Food Group

Food	Low GL (<10)	Medium GL (11–19)	High GL (>20)
Breads, crispbread	Whole-meal bread, 1 slice Rye bread, 1 slice Fruit bread, 1 slice	Crispbread, 2 Kavli, 3 Sao, Ryvita, 2 Crumpets, 2 Lebanese bread, 1 round	Bagel, 1 Croissant
Breakfast cereals	All Bran, 30 g (1 oz)	Rice Bubbles, 1 cup Puffed Wheat Sustain, Just Right Good Start Nutrigrain Porridge, 1 cup Special K (Australia and USA) Good Start, 2	
Pasta and rice		Spaghetti Ravioli Rice cakes, 2 Vermicelli, 1 cup	White rice, 1 cup Basmati rice, 1 cup
Vegetables, legumes	Swede Carrots, pumpkin Baked beans Beetroot	Instant potato, 1 cup Sweet potato Parsnip, 80 g (2.8 oz)	Baked potato, 1 medium Gnocchi, 1 cup
Fruit	Watermelon Rockmelon, canta-loupe Pineapple Mango, grapes, plums Orange Dried fruit	Banana	
Dairy foods	Ice cream, low fat, 1 scoop Ice cream, premium Milo on milk Flavoured milk, 250 mL (8 oz) Flavoured yogurt Milk—nonfat, full cream		
Snacks and confectionery	Plain biscuits, 2 M&Ms, 30 g (1 oz) Peanuts	Muesli bar Milk chocolate, 50 g (1.8 oz) Snickers	Jelly beans, 30 g (1 oz) Mars bar, 60 g (2 oz)
Sports drinks, soft drinks, fruit juice		Sports drink, 250 mL (8 oz) Fruit juice, 250 mL (8 oz)	Lucozade, 250 mL (8 oz) Fanta, 250 mL (8 oz) Coca-Cola, 250 mL (8 oz) Sustagen Sport, 250 mL (8 oz)
Sugars	Table sugar, 2 tsp		Glucose Glucodin

Adapted from S.K. Foster-Powell, H.A. Holt and J.C. Brand-Miller, 2002, "International table of glycemic index and glycemic load values: 2002," *Am J Clin Nutr* 76(1): 5-56. Adapted with permission by the *American Journal of Clinical Nutrition*. © Am J Clin Nutr. American Society for Clinical Nutrition.

FINAL SCORE

- Your muscles, your brain and your liver require carbohydrate (in the form of glucose) to function normally. Your body is a glucose-burning machine.

- If you eat too little carbohydrate, you are likely to tire quickly and not be able to sustain aerobic activity. A low-carbohydrate diet is by default a low-kilojoule diet, so you will lose weight but you won't be able to be active and you could be getting too little fibre, antioxidants and other essential nutrients.

- Carbohydrate supplements in the form of sports drinks, food bars or gels can provide useful additional carbohydrate for the very active endurance athlete. Snack foods and commercial liquid meals can help athletes reach their carbohydrate and nutrition goals in heavy training.

- Sugars are a normal part of the diet. They are not harmful, except when so much added-sugar foods are eaten that they displace other nutritious foods.

- Some sugar-containing foods are very nutritious, such as fruit, milk, yogurt, soy drinks and, believe it or not, chocolate.

- The glycemic index of food may be useful to some athletes. Moderate to high GI foods are quicker to digest, absorb and convert to glycogen than equal amounts of low GI foods. This could be an advantage to athletes training or competing more than once a day.

- The GI of a food may be of little advantage in meals before sport. It is probably more important that athletes eat enough great-tasting foods rich in carbohydrate, rather than focusing solely on the GI of foods and meals.

- Low GI foods generally are the least processed foods and are therefore more likely than high GI foods to have a reasonable level of nutrition and fibre.

four

Calcium, Iron and Vitamins for Health and Performance

> Some athletes may develop iron deficiency and this will impair performance. Calcium is important for healthy bones, especially in adolescents and in female athletes, so it is important to ensure adequate calcium intake.
>
> *Medical Commission of the International Olympic Committee (2004)*

This chapter focuses on some key vitamins and minerals that are of particular importance to active people. Of course, all vitamins and minerals are important, but several have particular benefits for athletes. Because iron deficiency will impede sports performance and poor bone strength will have long-term consequences, athletes should eat adequate iron and calcium. The vitamins that often get mentioned in sports performance are the B group vitamins as they are involved in energy production, and vitamins E and C as they are proposed to enhance performance.

Calcium

Calcium is an essential mineral that is part of the structure of teeth and bones. The body needs a daily supply of calcium for maximum bone strength throughout life. Our best sources of calcium are dairy foods (yogurt, milk and cheese—but not butter); calcium-fortified foods (e.g., some soy drinks) and the soft bones of canned sardines and salmon.

Osteoporosis and Physical Activity

Every day your bones are in a constant state of flux; some bone is manufactured and some is broken down as your bones are modeled and remodeled. Early in life, more bone is made than is broken down; hence, bones get bigger and stronger. Bone mass increases rapidly from puberty and peaks when people reach their 30s. Later in life the trend tends to be the opposite—more gets broken down than is formed, so bones become weaker.

If bones break down more quickly than they can be rebuilt, osteoporosis (brittle and weak bones) occurs, making them more likely to break as a result of minor injury. Postmenopausal women experience a more rapid breakdown of bone as a result of the drop in the female hormones estrogen and progesterone. (Estrogen prevents bone loss, whereas progesterone promotes bone formation.) Osteoporosis can occur in men too, although usually at a slower rate and at a later age than women. The best way to measure bone strength is by assessing bone mineral density (BMD): the lower the density, the greater the risk of bone fractures.

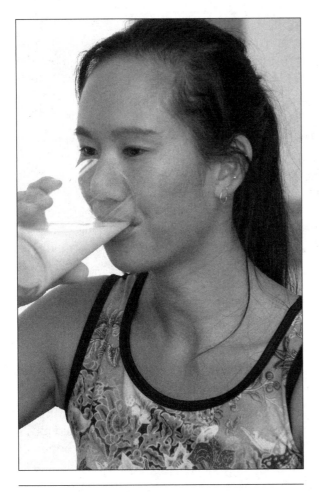

Daily calcium intake makes for strong bones.

Bones just love their exercise. Fitter people tend to have stronger bones, which is great for avoiding osteoporosis later in life. Weight-bearing exercise (e.g., running) is a wonderful stimulus to bone growth and strength as the skeleton adapts to the forces applied during running. Strength training will also apply

greater loads to the skeleton and can be effective in reducing bone loss, especially in the later years of life.

Weight-supported sports, such as cycling and swimming, are less effective at increasing bone mass as less force is applied to the skeleton. Most athletes, male and female, will have above-average bone mass and are less likely to get osteoporosis compared to those who do not get enough exercise in life.

Bone-Tired Women

If a female athlete has long and arduous training sessions, her menstrual pattern can become irregular and may even cease altogether (this is called amenorrhea). For some women this comes as a great relief—no more premenstrual syndrome. Unfortunately, having no periods means that the body is producing less estrogen, which stops bones from reaching their highest mass and strength. This less-than-normal amount of bone is called osteopenia, which may lead to osteoporosis. Nonmenstruating athletes tend to have a lower bone mass compared to the rest of the female population. Runners, especially distance runners, are more likely to stop having periods than are swimmers or team sport players.

Young amenorrheic females could be losing bone rather than building it, making them likely to suffer from stress fractures in the short term and premature osteoporosis in the long term. Because bone loss appears to be most rapid soon after periods stop, experts advise any athlete who stops menstruating for more than three months, or has very irregular periods, to see her doctor.

Factors That Increase the Risk of Osteoporosis

- Family history of osteoporosis
- Caucasian or Asian background
- Inadequate calcium in the diet
- Excessive amounts of dietary sodium (salt)
- Excessive caffeine
- Inactivity
- Cigarette smoking

Women only:
- Early menopause or ovary removal
- Amenorrhea

Remember that amenorrhea has other causes too, including not eating enough food (very strict diets), very low body weight and psychological stress. Amenorrheic athletes should check with a sports dietitian to ensure they are getting enough food to fuel performance and normal menstruation. Amenorrhea is also more likely to occur in women who had a history of irregular periods before they started heavy training.

As training becomes lighter, the amenorrhea is reversible and regular periods can return. Although more research needs to be done, it is heartening to note that bone loss can be reversed if periods recommence. Those involved in weight-bearing exercise seem to have greater protection against bone loss during amenorrhea than those in non-weight-bearing sports.

Calcium in Food

Too little dietary calcium has also been implicated as a cause of osteopenia and osteoporosis. More than 99 per cent of the body's calcium is found in bones and teeth. About 70 per cent of our calcium comes from the dairy foods milk, cheese and yogurt. Low-fat yogurt and milk are usually higher in calcium than the regular versions because when the fat is removed, manufacturers add back more milk solids, which includes calcium and protein. Around 20 per cent of all the calcium we eat is absorbed from our digestive system (mainly the duodenum, the first part of the small intestine). It is often said that we cannot absorb the calcium from milk, but in fact, we absorb around 30 per cent of the calcium from milk. Table 4.1 shows how much calcium you need each day, and table 4.2 lists the calcium content of some foods.

Calcium Supplements

For various reasons, some people choose not to eat dairy foods or calcium-fortified foods. If you believe you are not getting enough calcium from food, then taking a calcium supplement may be wise. Your doctor or dietitian can give you advice. If you take a supplement, check the label to see how much pure calcium you get, not the total amount of the calcium supplement. For example, 600 milligrams of calcium gluconate gives you only 55 milligrams of calcium, whereas 600 milligrams of calcium carbonate gives you about 250 milligrams of calcium, nearly five times as much. Calcium carbonate and calcium citrate are considered the better calcium supplements.

Iron

If you are very active, then you have an increased chance of becoming low in iron; your chance is increased if you are a young female.

Table 4.1   Daily Calcium Recommendations in Milligrams

		Australia/New Zealand	United States/ Canada	UK
Female				
Girls	9–13 yr	1,000	1,300	800
Teenagers	14–18 yr	1,300	1,300	800
Women	19–50 yr	1,000	1,000	700
Women	Pregnant	1,000	1,000	700
Women	Nursing	1,000	1,000	1,250
Women	51+ yr	1,300	1,200	700
Male				
Boys	9–13 yr	1,000	1,300	1,000
Teenagers	14–18 yr	1,300	1,300	1,000
Men	19–70 yr	1,000	1,000	700
Men	71+ yr	1,300	1,200	700

Table 4.2 Calcium Content of Some Common Foods

Food	Calcium (mg)
Milk and soy foods	
Calcium-fortified milk, 250 mL (8 oz)	500
Sustagen Sport, 200 mL (7 oz), with water	400
Nonfat milk, 250 mL (8 oz)	375
Reduced-fat (2% fat) milk, 250 mL (8 oz)	310
Low-fat (1% fat) milk, 250 mL (8 oz)	310
Flavoured milk, 250 mL (8 oz)	300
Calcium-fortified soy drink, 250 mL (8 oz)	300
Whole milk, 250 mL (8 oz)	275
Tofu, firm (calcium coagulant), 100 g (3.5 oz)	160
Tofu, soft (calcium coagulant), 100 g (3.5 oz)	80
Yogurt, per 200 g (7 oz)	
Low-fat, natural	360
Low-fat, fruit flavour	320
Plain, natural	290
Whole, fruit flavour	260
Cheese, per 30 g (1 oz)	
Edam	260
Cheddar	240
Processed	200
Camembert, Brie	150
Ricotta	100
Cottage cheese	30
Dairy desserts, per serve	
Frûche, low fat, 200 g (7 oz)	160
Custard, 100 mL (3 oz)	150
Ice cream, 1 scoop	65
Fat and oil, per serve	
Cream, 1 Tbsp	15
Butter, 1 Tbsp	5
Vegetable oils	0
Other foods, per serve	
Sardines + bones, 50 g (1.8 oz)	175
Molasses, blackstrap, 1 Tbsp	170
Collard, 1/2 cup cooked	170
Salmon + bones, 50 g (1.8 oz)	150
Prawns, 100 g (3.5 oz)	150
Spinach, 1/2 cup cooked	140
Milk chocolate, 50 g (1.8 oz)	125

Food	Calcium (mg)
Other foods, per serve	
Tahini, 1 Tbsp	90
Baked beans, 1 cup	90
Soybeans 1/2 cup	80
Bok choy, 1/2 cup cooked	80
Clams, 100 g (3.5 oz)	80
Almonds, 30 g (1 oz)	70
Kidney beans, chick peas, 1/2 cup	60
Brazil nuts, 30 g (1 oz)	55
Sesame seeds, 3 Tbsp, 30 g (1 oz)	40
Egg	35
Broccoli, 1 cup cooked	30
Dark chocolate, 50 g (1.8 oz)	25
Fruit juice, 250 mL (8 oz)	25
Fresh fruit, average	20
Bread, 1 slice	20
Peanuts, 30 g (1 oz)	20
Meat, chicken, 100 g (3.5 oz)	20
Peanut butter, 1 Tbsp	10
Pasta, 1 cup	10
Rice, 1 cup	5

Data sources include Nutrition information panels on food labels; Nutritional Values of Australian Foods. 1997. Canberra: Australian Government Publishing Service; U.S. Department of Agriculture, Agricultural Research Service. 2004. USDA National Nutrient Database for Standard Reference, Release 17. Nutrient Data Laboratory Home Page, http://www.nal.usda.gov/fnic/foodcomp.

Tips for Getting More Calcium Into Your Diet

- Change to nonfat or reduced-fat milk and low-fat yogurt; they generally have more calcium.
- Use low-fat milk in baking.
- Add yogurt or milk to soup, or a dab of yogurt to tacos, burritos and curries.
- Mix low-fat milk with mashed potato.
- Melt cheese on toast, baked potatoes or pasta dishes.
- If you don't like plain milk, blend it with fruit for a smoothie, or add some flavouring such as Milo, Nesquik, Aktavite, Ovaltine or Horlicks.
- Use commercial flavoured milks for a convenient snack. Most are made from reduced-fat milk.
- Eat green leafy vegetables such as broccoli, bok choy or Brussels sprouts as they have easy-to-absorb calcium. The exceptions are spinach and rhubarb, which have calcium in a form that is very difficult to absorb.
- If you don't eat dairy foods, choose a calcium-fortified soy beverage.
- Go easy on salt and salty foods. Too much salt in the diet may cause extra calcium to be lost in the urine. Choose reduced-salt varieties of food.
- Reduce caffeine intake. High levels of caffeine may reduce calcium absorption.

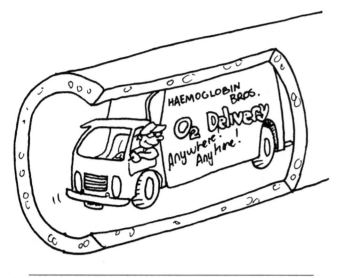

Figure 4.1 Iron is part of the hemoglobin protein complex found in blood. Hemoglobin collects oxygen to transport it to all cells in the body.

This section will discuss iron and how to avoid iron deficiency and its symptoms.

Most of the iron in the body is incorporated into hemoglobin, a protein in blood that takes oxygen from the lungs to all parts of the body and retrieves carbon dioxide from body cells to be exhaled (see figure 4.1). Iron is also found in myoglobin in muscles, which does a similar job to hemoglobin in that it stores oxygen. Iron is stored in ferritin molecules throughout the body. Some iron is lost from the body each day, and, ideally, the losses are replaced by eating iron-containing food.

Iron Depletion in Athletes

If iron losses are more than the iron absorbed by the digestive system, then body iron stores are gradually depleted. The first stage is called iron deficiency, where sports performance can drop, yet the athlete may not feel the more obvious symptoms of fatigue. Iron deficiency anemia occurs when all the body's iron stores have been used up and the athlete experiences constant fatigue. Iron depletion can occur in athletes when high-level exercise causes an increase in iron losses. Fortunately, anemia doesn't always follow because athletes can compensate for the extra iron losses by eating iron-rich food.

Most athletes suspect low iron levels when their training performance deteriorates despite putting in a good effort. If fatigue or poor performance persists and you suspect anemia, get a confirmation blood test from your doctor.

Symptoms of low iron include the following:

- Fatigue (for other causes of tiredness, see table 4.3)
- Listlessness
- Paler-than-normal skin
- Being more susceptible to infection (iron is needed for a healthy immune system)
- Decline in sports performance

Remember that many conditions can lead to fatigue. Note the serious warning below, and table 4.3, which lists possible causes of fatigue and their solutions.

Increased losses of iron from the body may occur in the following ways:

- **Via urine and feces.** Athletes tend to lose more iron this way than do other people. Blood loss from the stomach or the intestines seems to occur in endurance runners for reasons still unknown. It may be due to some minor damage caused by reduced blood flow to the intestinal lining as much of the blood is redirected to the

Serious Warning

Please do not take iron supplements if you are feeling a bit tired. About 1 in 250 people has an iron overload condition called hemochromatosis, whereby the body absorbs more iron than needed. It occurs in both men and women, although it is more common in men. Iron builds up in the liver, pancreas and heart, slowly destroying these organs. One of the symptoms is chronic tiredness. If you take an iron supplement in this situation, you will make things worse. See your doctor for a blood test if you are always tired. I know that 1 in 250 doesn't sound like many, but the consequences are dire as the liver, pancreas and heart are organs that are very difficult to repair or replace. Again, do not ever take iron supplements unless recommended by your doctor after a blood test.

Table 4.3   Fatigue Guide

Possible causes of fatigue	Solutions
Low iron levels	• Have a blood test. • Increase dietary iron. • Take iron supplements, if prescribed.
Too little carbohydrate	• Eat more carbohydrate foods and drinks, especially during heavy training programs. • Eat five or six times a day.
Overtraining or undertraining	• Reduce training. • Eat more carbohydrate-rich foods. • Check with your coach for a modified training schedule. • Lack of fitness can make people feel tired.
Gastric upset	• Don't eat too close to training; allow two hours or more between eating and exercise. • Drink plenty of fluids; avoid dehydration.
Too much caffeine	• Don't take caffeine close to bedtime. • Cut back on caffeine drinks such as high-caffeine 'energy' drinks.
Stress, worry	• Avoid the cause of stress. This may involve changing your job, your work hours, where you live, or relationships. • Learn relaxation techniques.
Dehydration	• Drink until you pass copious amounts of pale urine, especially after training.
Too much alcohol	• Reduce alcohol. • Explore why you need to drink unhealthy amounts.
Shiftwork	• This problem has no simple answer. It is best to get into a routine so that you sleep at the same time each day. • Enjoy light meals at work; don't overeat.
Premenstrual syndrome	• Reduce salt and salty foods; this can help reduce the bloated feeling.
Skipping meals	• Always eat regularly throughout the day, even if only for a light snack. Don't skip breakfast because that will make you tired and reduce your physical and mental performance. • Eat three to six times daily.
Study	• Fitting in study hours can be tough, especially if you work as well. Try to reshape the day by watching less TV and exercising every day.
Smoking	• The answer is obvious.
Hay fever, allergies	• See your doctor for the best advice to minimise symptoms. • Attend an allergy clinic at a major teaching hospital.
Timing of meals or snacks	• Leave two hours or more between eating and training. • Leave two hours or more between eating and going to bed. • Don't miss meals.
Overweight	• Lose body fat, especially abdominal fat.
Hypoglycemia	• Eat for health over five or six meals or snacks a day. • Note: Very few people have true hypoglycemia.
Weather	• Hot or humid weather can wipe you out until you acclimatise. • Train in the cooler part of the day if it is more comfortable. • Seek medical help if hay fever is a problem.

muscles in sport. It could also be due to the effects of some drugs such as aspirin.

Blood in the urine may be caused by minor damage to the lining of the bladder. It will usually clear up within 48 hours of strenuous exercise. Good hydration can reduce damage because having some urine in the bladder may lessen damage to the bladder lining. For most athletes, blood is not lost in this manner. See your doctor if you see blood in your urine or stools.

• **From running.** Every time the foot hits the ground during running, some red blood cells are destroyed, a process called hemolysis; hence it's called 'footstrike hemolysis'. This is not a problem for most athletes, but it can become an issue in endurance runners. Some of the hemoglobin released from the broken red blood cells may end up in the urine.

Check your running shoes and make sure they are well cushioned and that your running style is efficient. A sports podiatrist can help you here. If you are overweight, reduce your body fat stores to reduce the pressure on your feet.

• **Because of reduced iron absorption.** Normally, in most healthy people, the body compensates for low iron levels by absorbing more iron from food. This compensatory mechanism is sometimes blunted in athletes for reasons that are not clear.

• **From normal blood loss.** A good deal of iron can be lost during menstruation, which is the main reason young women need twice the iron as men. Blood can also be lost through injury and regular blood donations. I'm not suggesting that you stop being a blood donor, but you will have to consider when in your training schedule it is best to donate blood. One option is to be a plasma donor as you will then keep your red blood cells. For most active people, regular blood donations are not a problem, although you may want to take it easy on the day of the donation.

• **Via sweat.** Because athletes sweat more than sedentary people, it has been suggested that any iron losses in sweat could add up over months of heavy sweat loss such as during endurance training. This is unlikely to be a major cause of anemia in athletes.

Having noted all of the potential ways an athlete might lose more iron than normal, be aware that the most likely cause of iron deficiency anemia in athletes is menstrual loss in women and insufficient iron in the diet in both men and women.

Sports Anemia

Sports anemia is not a case of too little iron in the diet and therefore does not require an iron supplement. In sports anemia, ferritin and hemoglobin levels in the blood appear low, but this is due to the extra 10 to 20 per cent of plasma (the liquid part of blood) produced by athletes in heavy training. In other words, because there is more plasma, not less hemoglobin, hemoglobin levels only appear to be low.

Although the concentration of hemoglobin is lower in cases of sports anemia, the oxygen-carrying capacity of the blood is not affected. Sports anemia is sometimes impressively called dilutional pseudoanemia. The dilution makes the blood less viscous (less gluggy) so that blood can travel the blood vessel highways much more quickly, which is ideal for oxygen delivery to the muscles. The extra plasma may also help reduce the risk of dehydration. The dilution effect usually occurs early in a bout of increased training. The dilution reverses quickly over a few days if training ceases.

In some elite athletes extra red blood cells are made in response to training, which is also very useful in getting more oxygen to the muscles. Although there may be more red blood cells, there's an even larger increase in plasma, so dilutional pseudoanemia still occurs.

Blood Tests for Iron Deficiency and Anemia

A blood test is the best way to see whether an athlete has a true anemia. Blood should be taken on a rest day or before any strenuous exercise because dehydration will give falsely high readings as a result of the blood having become more concentrated. Table 4.4 lists the range of bloods tests for iron deficiency. In the laboratory, the blood is measured for the following:

• Serum iron (lower in iron deficiency)
• Total iron-binding capacity (TIBC) of the blood (higher in iron deficiency)
• Iron saturation of an iron-transporting protein called transferrin (the transferrin saturation level falls in iron deficiency)
• Concentration of ferritin (lower in iron deficiency)
• Hemoglobin level (lower in iron deficiency anemia)

Table 4.4   Blood Tests for Iron Deficiency

Blood test	Iron deficiency
Serum iron	<500 mcg/L
TIBC	>4,000 mcg/L
Transferrin saturation	<16%
Ferritin	<35 mcg/L
Hemoglobin	<120 g/L (12g/100mL)*

*A low hemoglobin level indicates that iron deficiency has now become clinical anemia.

When iron stores become depleted, the body can't make enough hemoglobin. This will lead to anemia and less oxygen being transported to muscles, which causes a deterioration in performance.

The measurement most widely used in sports medicine is that of plasma ferritin, a protein in which iron is stored. Iron is toxic to the body so it needs to be wrapped in the protective ferritin molecule. Ferritin is found mainly in the bone marrow, but a small amount of ferritin is found in the blood in proportion to the amount in the bone marrow. The range usually found in athletes is 30 to 200 micrograms per litre. A ferritin value below 15 micrograms per litre is considered to represent depleted bone marrow iron stores and is usually associated with fatigue and a decline in performance. Many sports physicians prescribe iron supplementation when the value is lower than 35 micrograms per litre.

The interpretation of ferritin levels is not straightforward. For example, smaller people, especially those with low muscle mass, have normally lower concentrations of ferritin and hemoglobin. Females have, on average, lower values than males have. A small female distance runner with a hemoglobin of 11 grams per 100 mL or a ferritin of 20 micrograms per litre may have near optimal levels. However, if a male weightlifter or footballer presented with these values, iron deficiency would be suspected. A sports physician is best placed to make a judgment on blood iron studies.

Who Is at Risk of Low Iron Stores?

The following types of people are at highest risk of having low iron stores:

- Male and female endurance runners as a result of footstrike hemolysis, greater iron loss in feces and urine, and extra iron losses from heavy sweating.

- Females with heavy periods. More blood loss means higher iron needs.

- Females on strict weight loss diets. Strict weight loss diets are generally low in many essential nutrients. It's very difficult to get all your iron needs when food is very restricted. When attempting body fat loss, choose low-fat foods high in iron, such as lean meat and iron-fortified breakfast cereals.

- Athletes avoiding iron-rich foods such as red meat, paté and iron-fortified foods, or avoiding foods high in vitamin C such as fruits and vegetables.

- Vegan athletes. Because they don't eat animal foods, they eat almost no easy-to-absorb iron.

Women are generally at greater risk of low iron as a result of menstrual losses and consuming less food than men. Very few men eat a low-iron diet.

Iron in Food

The iron in food is found in two different forms, heme and non-heme. Heme iron is well absorbed by the body (about 20 per cent is absorbed) and is found in animal flesh foods such as red meat, poultry and seafood. It is abundant in liver and kidney if you fancy that kind of fare. Non-heme iron is found in plant foods, but only around 5 per cent is absorbed.

The iron in spinach is poorly absorbed. (Popeye got it wrong!) Less than 2 per cent of the iron in spinach is absorbed because most of the iron is bound to natural compounds called oxalates and can't be absorbed by the intestines.

Cereal foods, vegetables and meat provide three quarters of the iron in a Western diet. There are around 6 to 7 milligrams of iron in every 4,200 kilojoules (1,000 cal) of food, which shows why women who have a restricted food intake have a greater risk of anemia. Use table 4.5 to check that there is enough iron in your meals.

Follow these tips to pump iron into your meals:

- **Include fruits or vegetables with each meal.** The vitamin C in fruits and vegetables enhances iron absorption, especially from other plant foods. A glass of orange juice with your breakfast cereal can nearly double your iron absorption.

Table 4.5   Daily Iron Recommendations in Milligrams

		Australia, New Zealand, United States, Canada	UK
Female			
Girls	9–13 yr	8	14.8
Teenagers	14–18 yr	15	14.8
Women	19–50 yr	18	14.8
Women	Pregnant	27	14.8
Women	Nursing	9	14.8
Women	51+ yr	8	8.7
Male			
Boys	9–13 yr	8	11.3
Teenagers	14–18 yr	11	11.3
Men	19+ yr	8	8.7

• **Eat lean red meat three or four times a week.** Red meat is your best source of easy-to-absorb iron. Poultry and fish also provide iron, although less than red meat.

• **Avoid drinking tea and coffee with meals.** The tannin in these drinks reduces iron absorption, by up to half. Drink tea between meals. Coffee contains less tannin than tea, but still needs to be considered as it has other compounds that reduce iron absorption.

• **Eat breakfast cereals.** Most breakfast cereals are fortified with iron. Check the label to see how much iron you get per serve. Because this is non-heme iron, you will need to take a vitamin C source with your cereal. Porridge and muesli are very nutritious, but they are not high in iron.

• **Avoid too much unprocessed bran.** Eat a maximum of two level tablespoons of bran daily. Avoid foods highly fortified with bran, as the bran can reduce iron absorption.

• **Take a low-dose multivitamin and mineral supplement.** They can be useful if you suspect you don't get enough iron and don't want to make dietary changes. Most will provide about 5 milligrams of iron per tablet. I strongly recommend that you see your doctor for a blood test before you take iron supplements.

Iron Supplements

If you think you suffer from low iron, ask your doctor to do a blood test to check. If iron deficiency is diagnosed, you will probably be prescribed an iron supplement for six weeks or longer to quickly get your iron levels back to normal. Naturally, you will also be advised to eat high-iron foods (see table 4.6).

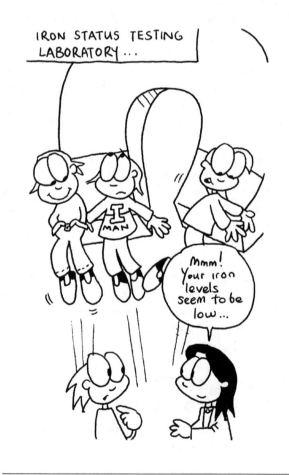

Are your iron levels too low?

Table 4.6 Iron Content of Some Common Foods

Food	Iron (mg)
Meats, seafood, egg	
Liver, 100 g (3.5 oz)	10.0
Lean beef, 100 g (3.5 oz)	3.8
Lean lamb, 100 g (3.5 oz)	3.5
Paté, 1 Tbsp	2.0
Lean pork, 100 g (3.5 oz)	1.0
Chicken leg, no skin, 100 g (3.5 oz)	1.0
Tuna, salmon, 100 g (3.5 oz)	1.0
Shellfish, av. serve	1.0
Egg, 1 whole	0.7
Chicken breast, no skin, 100 g (3.5 oz)	0.6
Fish, grilled, av., 100 g (3.5 oz)	0.6
Drinks	
Sustagen, 250 mL (8 oz)	4.0
Soy beverage, 250 mL (8 oz)	1.0
Milo, Ovaltine, 2 rounded tsp	1.0
Fruit juice, 250 mL (8 oz)	0.4
Milk	0.0
Breakfast cereals	
Weetbix Multi-Grain, 2 biscuits	3.0
Sportsplus, FibrePlus, 45 g (1.6 oz)	3.0
Cornflakes, 30 g (1 oz)	3.0
Just Right, Sustain, 30 g (1 oz)	3.0
Iron-fortified cereals, 45 g (1.6 oz)	2.5+
Weetbix, 2 biscuits	2.5
Breakfast bars, 1 average	2.5
Sultana Bran, 30 g (1 oz)	2.0
Muesli, 1/2 cup	1.5
Vita Brits, 2 biscuits	1.0
Porridge, 3/4 cup	1.0
Wheat germ, 1 Tbsp	0.6
Breads, rice and pasta	
Whole-meal bread, 1 slice	0.6
Fruit loaf, 1 slice	0.6
White bread, 1 slice	0.4
Pasta, 1/2 cup	0.4
Rice, 1/2 cup	0.3

(continued)

Table 4.6 *(continued)*

Food	Iron (mg)
Vegetables, fruits, nuts, seeds	
Spinach, 100 g (3.5 oz)	3.0
Baked beans, lentils, kidney beans, 1/2 cup	2.0
Cashews, 30 g (1 oz)	1.5
Peas, 1/2 cup	1.3
Dried apricots, 5 pieces	1.3
Almonds, 30 g (1 oz)	1.0
Potato, 1 medium	0.8
Sunflower seeds, 1 Tbsp	0.8
Raisins, 2 Tbsp	0.6
Vegetables, av. serve	0.5
Fresh fruit, 1 serve	0.5
Peanuts, 30 g (1 oz)	0.5
Peanut butter, 1 Tbsp	0.5
Confectionery, muesli bars	
Licorice, 50 g (1.8 oz)	4.0
Muesli bars, 1 av.	2.0
Dark chocolate, 50 g (1.8 oz)	1.5
Milk chocolate, 50 g (1.8 oz)	0.7

Vitamins

There are 13 different compounds considered as vitamins. These are conveniently divided into two groups, water soluble (B group vitamins and vitamin C) and fat soluble (vitamins A, D, E and K). Vitamins were one of the earliest supplements to be given to athletes, yet more than 40 years later there is no definite proof that extra vitamins actually improve performance, except in the rare athlete who has a clear vitamin deficiency.

An athlete making wise food choices is very unlikely to find a benefit in a vitamin supplement. Researchers from the Australian Institute of Sport gave 82 athletes a vitamin and mineral supplement for seven months and concluded, 'This study provided little evidence of any effect of supplementation to athletic performance for athletes consuming the dietary Recommended Dietary Intakes' (Telford 1992). They further commented that part of the reason Russian laboratories find a performance benefit with vitamin supplements is the fact that a lack of fresh fruits and vegetables in parts of Russia can lead to vitamin deficiency. Furthermore, the American College of Sports Medicine stated, 'In general, no vitamin and mineral supplements should be required if an athlete is consuming adequate energy from a variety of foods to maintain body weight' (American College of Sports Medicine 2000).

B Group Vitamins

The B vitamins thiamin (B_1), riboflavin (B_2), niacin (B_3) and pantothenic acid (B_5) are involved in the metabolism of carbohydrate and fat. Pyridoxine (B_6), folate and cyanocobalamin (B_{12}) are involved in making red blood cells. An increased need for these vitamins could be expected in athletes. Because training generally increases appetite, more food is eaten, providing extra B vitamins to meet those increased needs. Table 4.7 lists food sources for the B vitamins.

Table 4.7   Good Sources of B Vitamins

Food	Amount
Foods with thiamin (B$_1$)	
Hazelnuts, 50 g (1.8 oz)	0.2 mg
Sweet corn, cooked, 1/2 cup	0.2 mg
Peas, cooked, 1/2 cup	0.2 mg
Bread, whole meal, 1 slice	0.1 mg
Foods with riboflavin (B$_2$)	
Milk, low fat, 250 mL (8 oz)	0.5 mg
Yogurt, low fat, 200 g (7 oz)	0.4 mg
Almonds, 50 g (1.8 oz)	0.4 mg
Chicken, roasted 100 g (3.5 oz)	0.3 mg
Foods with niacin (B$_3$)	
Ham, lean, 100 g (3.5 oz)	8 mg
Mushroom, 100 g (3.5 oz)	4 mg
Banana, 1 medium	1 mg
Bread, whole meal, 1 slice	0.7 mg
Foods with pantothenic acid (B$_5$)	
Pork roast, 120 g (4.2 oz)	1.2 mg
Avocado, 100 g (3.5 oz)	1 mg
Milk, 250 mL (8 oz)	1 mg
Egg, boiled, 60 g (2 oz)	1 mg
Foods with pyridoxine (B$_6$)	
Banana, 1 medium	0.4 mg
Tuna, canned, 120g (4.2 oz)	0.4 mg
Beef, cooked, 120 g (4.2 oz)	0.3 mg
Peanuts, raw, 50 g (1.8 oz)	0.2 mg
Foods with folate	
Folate-fortified breakfast cereals, av. serve	100 mcg
Legumes such as kidney beans, cooked, 1/2 cup	100 mcg
Cabbage, cooked, 1/2 cup	40 mcg
Mushroom, 100 g (3.5 oz)	40 mcg
Foods with cyanocobalamin (B$_{12}$)	
Liver, cooked, 100g (3.5 oz)	70 mcg
Sardines, canned, 60g (2 oz)	14 mcg
Beef, cooked, 120g (4.2 oz)	2 mcg
Egg, boiled, 60 g (2 oz)	1 mcg

One of the B vitamins can be a detriment to performance. High-dose supplements of niacin or nicotinic acid (around 1,000 mg) can slow down an endurance athlete. Normally the body uses a mix of fat and glycogen as fuels. Niacin keeps the body from using fat as a fuel source so the body then has to rely heavily on glycogen for fuel. Because glycogen runs out quickly, the athlete 'hits the wall' earlier in the event.

Vitamin B_{12} is necessary for making DNA (the genetic director in body cells), so it has been hypothesised that it may stimulate muscle growth. However, there is no evidence that B_{12} will increase muscle growth or strength.

Vitamin E

Vitamin E is the common name for eight related compounds comprising four tocopherols and four tocotrienols. Of these, alpha-tocopherol is the most biologically active and the most widely distributed in food. The vast majority of studies since 1955 have reported no useful effect of vitamin E on improving sports performance. It also appears that the practice of vitamin E supplementation is not harmful, although an upper intake limit has been set at 300 milligrams daily. Table 4.8 lists food sources of vitamin E.

Vitamin C

Vitamin C assists the absorption of iron and has antioxidant activity. Early reports of vitamin C improving sports performance in Eastern European athletes was probably due to correcting a vitamin C deficiency caused by a lack of fruits and vegetables in the diet. Around 100 to 200 milligrams of vitamin C daily will saturate the body's cells, and extra amounts are unlikely to assist the athlete given that this amount is easily

Table 4.8 Good Sources of Vitamin E

Food	Amount (mg)
Almonds, 30 g (1 oz)	7.3
Mixed nuts, 30 g (1 oz)	3.1
Safflower oil, 1 Tbsp	3.6
Avocado, 1/2	2.1

Table 4.9 Good Sources of Vitamin C

Food	Amount (mg)
Red capsicum/red pepper, 1/2 cup	140
Orange, 1 medium	70
Broccoli, cooked, 1/2 cup	35
Pineapple, 1/2 cup	30

Data sources include *Nutritional Values of Australian Foods.* 1997. Canberra: Australian Government Publishing Service; U.S. Department of Agriculture, Agricultural Research Service. 2004. USDA National Nutrient Database for Standard Reference, Release 17. Nutrient Data Laboratory Home Page, http://www.nal.usda.gov/fnic/foodcomp.

obtained by eating fresh fruits and vegetables. For example, as you can see from table 4.9, one medium orange provides about 70 milligrams of vitamin C.

Although vitamin C does act as an antioxidant, the body responds to training by producing more of its own antioxidants. For this reason, taking extra vitamin C as a supplement doesn't seem to offer performance benefits. Indeed, oversupplementation can diminish the body's natural immune system.

Vitamin Supplements

Any athlete greatly restricting food intake or fasting to lose weight is probably getting too few vitamins. Athletes at most risk would be gymnasts, ballet dancers and anyone in a weight-restricted sport. If you are travelling to a country with a reputation for low-quality food (e.g., poor food safety or variety), then a vitamin supplement may be useful. Someone eating very little food may benefit from a low-dose multivitamin supplement, but megadosing has no value.

Clearly, the relationship between vitamins and sports performance needs further investigation. Most research will not be able to pick up a 0.5 or 1.0 per cent improvement in performance. Very little has been done to study the effect of vitamin supplements on recovery or injury prevention in elite athletes. Some vitamins in some athletes in certain conditions could make a small, but useful, difference in performance. There is a small amount of evidence that vitamin C and B complex supplements may help athletes get used to hot conditions and that vitamin E may help performance at high altitudes, but more research is needed.

If you truly believe you need a vitamin supplement, then get an inexpensive, low-dose supplement and avoid the popular high-dose, high-priced supplements. Check your vitamin supplement against the recommended amounts needed each day detailed in chapter 1. Providing more than is recommended is probably wasteful. Your diet should be providing the recommended amounts or more.

Taking a vitamin supplement is unlikely to cause any harm, but, as any sports dietitian will remind you, a vitamin supplement should never be a substitute for good eating habits.

Vitamin O

Supplements of stabilised oxygen molecules in a solution of sodium chloride and distilled water have been promoted. This supplement is supposed to treat everything from mild fatigue to cancer, heart problems and lung disease. It is being promoted to athletes as a tonic. It is also a big hoax.

Although it is called vitamin O, oxygen is not a vitamin, and nor is it something deficient in your diet. This is the world's most expensive salty water. Even if the water were as high in oxygen as claimed, it would help only if you were a fish breathing through gills.

The oxygen content of your glass of tap water is around 8 milligrams per litre. If you pressurise the water with oxygen gas, that level might increase to 40 milligrams per litre or more. When you open the bottle of 'vitamin O', most of this extra oxygen is released. In comparison, 1 litre of air contains 146 milligrams of oxygen, and when that runs out, golly, take another breath. Humans take oxygen from their lungs, not their intestines. Give 'vitamin O' a big miss.

FINAL SCORE

- Exercise in general will improve the strength and density of bones. Weight-bearing exercise, such as walking, aerobics, running, netball, football and strength training, offer the greatest protection against osteoporosis.
- Eating a diet rich in calcium reduces the risk of osteoporosis. Avoid excessive amounts of salt and caffeine as they may trigger calcium loss from the body.
- Low levels of iron are common in athletes and young women.
- Female athletes with amenorrhea for more than three months should see their doctor and a sports dietitian.
- An inadequate amount of iron in the diet is common in young women, vegans, vegetarians and those on restricted weight loss diets.
- Iron supplements should never be taken unless a doctor has diagnosed an iron deficiency.
- To minimise the risk of low iron intake, eat foods high in heme iron; otherwise, if vegetarian, consume foods containing vitamin C with each meal to enhance iron absorption
- Most athletes can get all their vitamin needs from food. A low-dose vitamin supplement will probably do no harm, but it should not be a substitute for good eating habits.

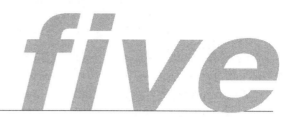

Liquids for Hydration, Cooling and Energy

Dehydration decreases exercise performance; thus, adequate fluid before, during, and after exercise is necessary for health and optimum performance. Athletes should drink enough fluid to balance their fluid losses.

American College of Sports Medicine
(2000)

Dehydration and heat stress continue to be major causes of poor sports performance, especially in warm weather. Athletes consider dehydration to be like pregnancy—either you are or you aren't. In fact, performance can decline very early in sport, well before you start to feel thirsty and tired. Dehydration will reduce muscle endurance, aerobic capacity and mental function. In the United States there is an average of three deaths a year from dehydration in American football players. In 1997 three U.S. college wrestlers died after using dehydration as a weight loss strategy.

Public interest in this topic was spurred when Gabriela Andersen-Schiess showed the classic signs of dehydration and heatstroke as she finished the first women's Olympic mara-

thon in 1984. Her legs had lost all coordination. At times she was on all fours, and yet the crowd pleaded—no, insisted—that she make the finish line. The 75,000 spectators created a heroine, and the TV producer loved every rating minute. But sports physicians were furious. Those who saw the image of the staggering athlete will likely never forget it.

Heat Stress

This chapter explains how to avoid heat stress, which includes the heat-related problems of heat exhaustion and heatstroke. Heat exhaustion is a condition in which the body starts to have difficulty maintaining a healthy core temperature. As the ability of the body to lose heat becomes lower than the amount of heat produced by exercise, the body's core temperature begins to rise and performance begins to drop. The symptoms of heat exhaustion are as follows:

- Nausea and vomiting
- Headache
- Faintness
- Profuse sweating

If you ever experience these symptoms, sit in the shade, drink lots of fluid and stop exercising for the rest of the day. If you were to continue exercising, you would likely go to the next stage, the extremely dangerous heatstroke. Heatstroke is a life-threatening condition in which the body temperature rises dangerously high, with sports performance dropping rapidly.

The symptoms of heatstroke include the following:

- Dizziness
- Nausea
- Cramps
- Headache
- Reduced sweating (due to lack of body fluids)
- Hot, dry skin

Although you may not be aware of it as it is happening, if you have these symptoms, you may be in urgent need of medical attention. People suffering from the flu or fever, and those who are overweight, not acclimatised to hot conditions or drink alcohol during the day before the event, are more susceptible to heat stress.

Temperature Regulation

To perform at your best, you will need to keep your body from overheating. The three main ways the body can lose the heat generated by muscle contraction during sport are illustrated in figure 5.1 and explained in more detail in this section.

- **Conduction.** When two objects at different temperatures come into contact with each other, heat will transfer from the hotter object to

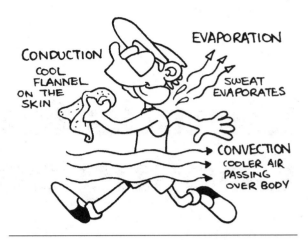

Figure 5.1 Heat transfer during sport.

the cooler object. For example, when an athlete runs on a hot road, heat is transferred from the road to the shoes and feet. Being sprayed with cold water can bring relief to the hot athlete as heat is transferred from the body to the water. The loss of too much heat is also common in long-distance open-water swimmers as the water is cooler than the body.

- **Convection.** Convection occurs when heat is transferred from the body to air when the air is much cooler than the body. As air moves across the skin, the warm air on the surface of the skin is replaced by cool air. This is especially effective in windy conditions. This method of heat loss is well known to the snow skier or cyclist coming down a hill. When a cold wind is blowing (the wind chill factor), it can be a bit too cool and you'll need to wear warmer clothing to prevent hypothermia.

- **Evaporation.** Evaporative cooling is the most important cooling method available to

City to Surf

The annual City to Surf fun run in Sydney, Australia, attracts over 40,000 participants. Although it is usually held in cool August conditions, runners still suffer from dehydration and heat exhaustion. After two runners died of heatstroke in 1990, the medical directors of the City to Surf surveyed the runners. The survey revealed that the four major risk factors for heat exhaustion were as follows (Lyle et al. 1994):

- Being highly motivated to do a personal best
- Not including at least one training session a week at the time the run is scheduled, to help acclimatise for the run
- Failing to drink fluids during the run
- Having a previous history of heat exhaustion

most athletes. About 70 per cent of body heat is lost when sweat evaporates and the liquid water is converted to water vapour. If the day is humid, this method becomes less effective because with more moisture in the air it becomes more difficult to evaporate sweat from the skin. Sweat that rolls off the skin is not being evaporated and has very little cooling effect.

Sweat It Out

During exercise, muscles use the energy from ATP to contract. Only 25 per cent of energy is actually used for muscle contraction. The other 75 per cent is released as heat. So that our muscles don't overheat and 'melt', the heat is transferred to blood. Our clever bodies then increase the blood flow to the skin so this heat can be released from the warmed blood by evaporative cooling (sweating), convection (breeze) and conduction (cooler ambient temperature).

Sweating from your many sweat glands is a very effective way of keeping your body cool. In fact, it's so good that as you get fitter, you will sweat more. As shown in figure 5.2, sweat originates from the water in your blood. Your heart was pumping around every bead of sweat on your brow at one time. Sweat fills your sweat glands, to be released once things get warm. The sweat on the surface of your skin will then evaporate to cool you down. If 1 litre of sweat fully evaporates from the skin, it dissipates 2,400 kilojoules (580 cal) of heat.

As you sweat, the water level in your blood begins to drop. As your blood volume drops, less blood flows to the skin, which further hinders heat loss. When dehydration is extreme and too much blood volume is lost, the body

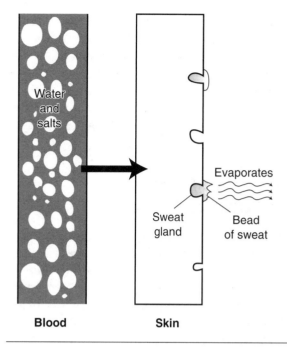

Figure 5.2 Sweat comes from the blood. More water than salt is lost from the blood during sweating.

stops sweating to preserve the remaining blood volume. Unfortunately, the body temperature quickly rises, and you will suffer heatstroke.

Sweat Glands

There are two types of sweat glands: eccrine and apocrine. The estimated 2 to 5 million eccrine sweat glands are all over your body, with the main concentration being on the palms of your hands and the soles of your feet. They produce an odour-free mix of water, sodium, potassium and chloride, with a single purpose—cooling the body.

Keeping Cool During Exercise

- Avoid sunburn. Apart from the discomfort, sunburned skin sweats less efficiently.
- Wear light-coloured and loose clothing.
- Avoid exercise in the heat of the day.
- Avoid dehydration—drink plenty of fluids.
- Apply cool water to the neck and head regions for cooling.
- Don't use oil-based sunscreens as these will interfere with evaporative cooling.
- Be fit. Unfit people are at greater risk of heatstroke.

Apocrine sweat glands are situated in the armpits and groin region. These glands produce fat, proteins and various steroids and secrete them into the base of hair follicles. The yellowish fluid has no smell, but bacteria on your skin will consume the secretions, producing a range of malodorous compounds. The smell of sweat is actually bacteria excrement. Ugh!

How Much Does an Athlete Sweat?

Most athletes will sweat at 500 to 1,000 mL per hour. (Remember that 1,000 mL is 1 litre.) This will be higher in hot conditions, when an athlete can easily lose 1 to 2 litres each hour, and it's difficult to replace that amount during the event.

The stomach empties at around 1,000 to 1,200 mL an hour, but athletes tend to drink much less than that. Research on runners shows that they drink 500 mL (17 oz) or less each hour, while sweating at 1,000 to 1,500 mL per hour. The volume that most athletes drink voluntarily during exercise is less than a half of their fluid losses. With training and encouragement athletes can drink 1,000 mL each hour (see figure 5.3). Fluids taken in sport are absorbed back into the blood to return the blood volume to normal, keeping

proper blood flow to the skin, which in turn helps sweating and prevents excessive heat buildup in the body.

Sometimes you won't notice yourself sweating. If you exercise in warm, dry conditions, the sweat can evaporate so quickly that you don't appear to be sweating. A good example is bike riding. As your body moves through the air, sweat evaporates almost as quickly as it's produced. In a sport like swimming, in which you are constantly wet, it is very difficult to work out how much you have sweated. Yes, you still sweat when you swim. A study of the swimmers at the Australian Institute of Sport in warm conditions found that 100 to 150 mL (3 to 5 oz) of fluid was lost for every kilometre swum (Cox et al. 2002). Being immersed in water will also suppress the thirst sensation; hence, dehydration may go unnoticed in activities such as swimming and water polo.

Men, Women and Children

Generally, women lose less sweat than men do. It's probably because they are more economical in their sweating and, because of their lower body weight, produce less sweat for the same workload. However, women appear to be as effective as men in 'keeping their cool' during exercise in the heat.

Children are at greater risk of overheating than adults are for the following reasons:

- Their sweating is less efficient so they depend more on convection for heat loss.
- Their ability to transfer heat from the centre of the body to the surface of the body (skin) by blood is less than that of adults.
- They produce more heat per kilogram at a given running speed.
- They have a larger surface area to body mass ratio than adults so can gain heat faster on hot days.

Therefore, even when topped up with fluids, children are at much greater risk of heatstroke than are adults. Unfortunately, children, like adults, don't drink enough fluids during exercise in the heat; frequent drink breaks should be encouraged.

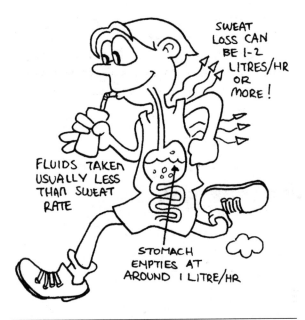

SWEAT LOSS CAN BE 1-2 LITRES/HR OR MORE!

FLUIDS TAKEN USUALLY LESS THAN SWEAT RATE

STOMACH EMPTIES AT AROUND 1 LITRE/HR

Figure 5.3 In warm weather, train yourself to drink at least 1 litre of fluid every hour.

Do You Need Extra Salt?

Sweat does contain sodium (salt), so as you sweat, you will lose sodium from the body. This is of little concern to most athletes training or competing for 90 minutes or less. The sodium losses will be replaced by sodium taken in a sports drink or in the next snack or meal.

If sweat losses are heavy over a day of physical activity or working in hot conditions, then it is possible that too much sodium can be lost, leading to muscle cramps. The sports drink with its extra sodium can be a very useful ally in replacing sodium losses during activity. Don't take salt tablets, as these are a very concentrated source of sodium and tend to suck fluid from the blood and into the small intestine, possibly causing abdominal pain. (See also the section on cramps on page 83.)

The Thirst Response

In most circumstances, when your body water levels drop, your body triggers a feeling of thirst and you will replace the lost water. Thirst is a very good indicator of your fluid needs during the day around the home or office and while doing daily chores. During sport and working in hot conditions, however, you can be dehydrated without feeling thirsty. There is no doubt that athletes should start drinking long before they become thirsty. Athletes can lose 2 per cent of their body weight as fluid (1.4 kg, or 1.4 L, in a 70 kg or 154 lb person) before experiencing the thirst sensation. This delay is called *voluntary dehydration* even though it is not a result of conscious behaviour. If you feel thirsty during training or sport, you are definitely getting too little fluid and will have difficulty catching up on fluid losses during exercise.

You can be dehydrated without feeling thirsty. Athletes should start drinking long before they become thirsty.

It was once thought that drinking during an event was a sign of weakness, especially in male sports. Even marathoners weren't allowed to drink before the 11-kilometre mark up until 1977. You cannot 'train' your body to cope with dehydration. Coaches who suggest training on little fluid to toughen the body are handing out very old-fashioned advice that could be dangerous. We now appreciate that chronic dehydration can occur in athletes who train frequently without topping up their fluid losses every day.

Remember: Weight loss during exercise is mainly sweat loss and needs to be replaced. Although some fat is used during exercise, it's not likely to be more than 50 grams in a 90-minute session. That's not to imply that exercise doesn't assist the loss of body fat. Evidence suggests that exercise is valuable in weight control by helping to 'normalise' your appetite (see chapter 12).

Acclimatisation

If you're going from a cool environment to a warm environment, it is smart to acclimatise to the local conditions for 10 to 14 days before competition (providing you have the time, of course). Exercising in local conditions hastens acclimatisation. If you travel across multiple time zones, you will ideally need around a week just to acclimatise to the new time zone.

When you acclimatise to warmer weather, several things happen:

- Extra blood is produced (up to 12 per cent more) so there is sufficient blood to supply both the exercising muscles and direct blood to the skin for cooling.

- You start sweating earlier and at a lower body temperature.

- You produce more sweat to maximise evaporative cooling (therefore, you will need more fluids).

- You lose less salt (sodium) in your sweat, reducing your risk of sodium-depletion cramps in long events.

Hyponatremia: Can You Drink Too Much Water?

There have been recorded cases of ultra-endurance athletes drinking more fluid than they lose as sweat and getting low blood sodium (hyponatremia), resulting in confused thinking, incoordination and weakness. In severe cases, people have died: Seven deaths of ultra-endurance athletes and military personnel from hyponatremia were recorded up to 2004, usually when they drank more water than they lost through sweating. This most commonly occurs in exercise taking longer than four hours.

As athletes sweat, they lose both electrolytes (e.g., sodium and potassium) and water. If, over a few hours, they replace just the water through drinking and not the sodium, the level of sodium drops in the blood. The body thinks there is too much water in the blood and transfers some water out of the blood and into other parts of the body, such as the brain. The brain begins to swell, hence the confused thinking and incoordination.

Hyponatremia is uncommon, as someone would have to drink a lot of water over many hours to cause this. For most athletes, including endurance athletes, excess fluid is passed via the bladder and fluid overload is rarely a problem; drinking too little is a greater hazard.

Those at greatest risk of hyponatremia are ultra-endurance athletes in mild weather conditions who take a long time to complete the course, while drinking plenty of water, such as someone who takes over four hours to finish

a 42-kilometre (26-mile) marathon. If you are involved in ultra-endurance events, take a sports drink as they have added sodium, and make sure your snacks and meals have sodium. It is partly for this reason that sports drinks contain sodium at 20 to 50 milligrams per 100 mL to assist the replacement of sodium lost in sweat. If you replace only water and not sodium during long periods of sweating, the concentration of plasma sodium can become dangerously low. Consult a sports dietitian for advice if you are into ultra-endurance sports.

There have been cases of water intoxication, but only after drinking vast amounts of water. In 1999, a 19-year-old U.S. Air Force recruit collapsed during a 10-kilometre (6-mile) walk. Doctors say it was the result of hyponatremia and heatstroke. In 2000, a 20-year-old U.S. Army recruit drank over 12 litres of water in an estimated 3-hour period. She lost consciousness and died from swelling in the brain and lungs from hyponatremia. Then in March 2002, a 19-year-old U.S. Marine died from drinking too much water during a 42-kilometre (26-mile) march (Gardner 2002). It is thought that overzealous instructors, not wanting a heatstroke or dehydration victim under their command, pushed the drinking of water to the limit.

To minimise the chance of hyponatremia, the message to endurance athletes is as follows:

- Drink fluids frequently.
- Do not drink more than you sweat.
- Choose sports drinks as your main fluid.

Cricketers Caught Behind on Fluids

Australian researchers studied 20 male first-grade cricket players (8 batsmen, 12 bowlers; average age 19 years) under both real match and simulated match conditions and at different temperatures (Gore, Bourdon, Woolford and Pederson 1993). Under cool conditions (22 °C or 72 °F) the players sweated at an average of 540 mL per hour, in warm conditions (30 °C or 86 °F) at 700 mL per hour, and in hot conditions (38 °C or 100 °F) at 1,370 mL per hour. Three bowlers on the hot day peaked at a sweat loss of 1,670 mL per hour.

During the cool day and the warm day, dehydration was 0.3 per cent and 1.2 per cent, respectively, which suggests that the current drink break schedule (one break each hour) is adequate under these conditions.

But after two sessions of play on the hot day, the average dehydration of the three fast bowlers was a loss of 4.3 per cent (3 kg in a 70 kg person; 6.7 lb in a 155 lb person) of their starting body weight despite drinking over 2.5 litres of fluid in that time. There is no doubt that this fluid loss compromised their performance.

The researchers stated, 'The implication for cricket is that skill levels, and therefore performance, will diminish as dehydration increases beyond 2% of initial body weight' (Gore, Bourdon, Woolford and Pederson 1993, p. 387).

Now, in international Test matches and one-day matches, it is possible for cricketers to get a sports drink or water from a drink bucket on the boundary or from an underground receptacle behind the wickets.

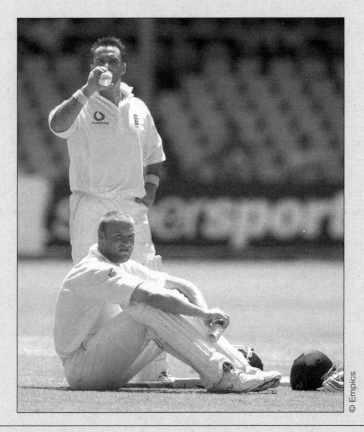

Cricket is a summer sport, making cricketers prone to dehydration. Breaks in play are a great opportunity to replace fluids lost as sweat.

That's Hot!

In December 1987, cricket batsman Allan Border lost 5 kilograms (11 lb) during a mammoth innings in a cricket Test match against New Zealand at the Adelaide Oval. He scored 205 (599 minutes) in official temperatures of 40.7 °C (105 °F).

Dehydration and Sports Performance

Dr. Lawrence Armstrong, Ball State University, assessed the effect of dehydration on running (Armstrong, Costill and Fink 1985). Running speed was reduced by 6 to 7 per cent with just a 2 per cent decrease in body weight from fluid loss. Even a 1 per cent reduction in body weight added an extra 17 seconds to a 1,500-metre run time. For the serious athlete, that could mean the difference between first place and a huge disappointment. In the 1996 Olympic men's marathon only eight seconds separated the gold medal winner and the bronze medallist, a mere 0.1 per cent difference in performance!

Another study by Dr. R.M. Walsh (Walsh et al. 1994) at the University of Cape Town

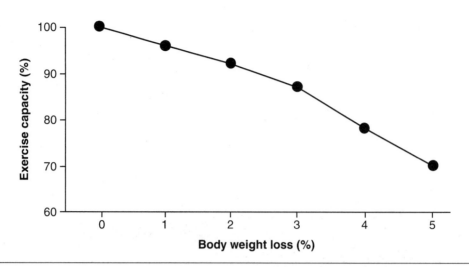

Figure 5.4 The effects of dehydration on performance can begin early.

From A. Jeukendrup and M. Gleeson, 2004, *Sport Nutrition: An Introduction to Energy Production and Performance*, page 177, figure 8.5. ©2004 by Human Kinetics Publishers. Reprinted with permission from Human Kinetics.

Medical School found that a 1.8 per cent drop in body weight during exercise affected sprint performance after 60 minutes of exercise. In practical terms this means that even low levels of dehydration can affect performance near the end of most team games and endurance events. As a general rule, there is a 5 per cent drop in sports performance for every 1 per cent drop in body weight (see figure 5.4).

Drinking Schedule

Here is an approximate fluid replacement schedule for sport. It will vary depending on the temperature of the venue, your sweat rate and your level of fitness. Use it as a guide only.

Before Sport

Drink 300 to 500 mL (two to three glasses) in the 15 minutes before exercise. This is your 'reserve' fluid. Although you will not feel thirsty at the time of drinking, this fluid is being absorbed into your blood at the same time you begin to sweat at the start of your sport. For many athletes, especially endurance athletes, this is the most important drink break.

During Sport

Drink 150 to 250 mL (5 to 8 oz) every 15 minutes, or at suitable breaks in sport. The stomach can empty at 1,000 to 1,200 mL per hour, and in warm weather it is ideal to drink at a similar rate. Even in cool weather, athletes can sweat 1 litre or more per hour.

After Sport

Drink to replace all lost fluids during sport, plus another 25 to 50 per cent because some of that fluid will be lost as urine. This means that you will need to drink at least 500 mL (17 oz) and probably a lot more if you have lost a lot of sweat. To determine how much fluid you have lost, you can use the weigh-in method described next.

Dehydration

Several studies have demonstrated a decreased stomach emptying rate with hypohydration (reduced body fluid levels) and hyperthermia. That means that when you are dehydrated, less fluid is being absorbed to replace fluid losses. This is a reminder to start drinking early in sport. Anxiety associated with sport (e.g., finals) can also greatly reduce the gastric emptying rate.

Check Your Water Level

There's a simple way to check your fluid loss during training sessions and events. Weigh yourself before and after training or competition. If possible, weigh yourself nude, otherwise in minimal clothing (so you are not weighing the sweat lost into your clothing). Although they are not usually accurate in displaying your body weight, bathroom scales will give you a good idea of total weight loss. Ideally, you should be drinking enough fluids to replace most sweat losses during the event. In my experience it is common for footballers, basketballers and other athletes to lose 2 to 4 per cent of their body weight during competition.

To determine your percentage of weight loss, use the following formula:

$$\frac{(\text{Presport weight}) - (\text{postsport weight}) \times 100}{\text{Presport weight}}$$

For example, if you are a 70-kilogram person who lost 1.4 kilograms (i.e., 1.4 litres overall fluid loss) in a training session,

$$\frac{(70 \text{ kg} - 68.6 \text{ kg}) \times 100}{70 \text{ kg}} = 2\% \text{ body weight loss}$$

Whatever weight you have lost during sport needs to be immediately replaced by fluids even if you don't feel thirsty. You will need to actually drink more than your fluid losses as not all the fluid you drink after sport will be retained by the body. Some will end up as urine. So the person in the previous example would need to drink more than 2,000 mL of fluid to replace his or her fluid loss.

Athletes who do a lot of training may be dehydrated before they start exercise, so their pretraining weight could be less than ideal. For those training a lot, I recommend that you take your nude weight every morning. If you see differences of more than 1 kilogram (2.2 lb), then you are likely to be starting the day dehydrated. For example, one rower I advised started the day between 77 and 79 kilograms. He thought the difference was fat loss and was disappointed when I told him that 79 kilograms was his true weight and 77 kilograms was a dehydrated weight.

Is That Clear-ish?

A simple guide to your fluid levels is the colour of your urine. As a general rule, if it is pale yellow or clear, you're well hydrated. If it is dark orange, you need to drink more fluids now. If you can't remember the last time you had a pee, you desperately need fluids.

The colour of your urine is not always a good indicator of hydration. After high sweat losses, you can still produce clear urine even when still dehydrated. How can this happen? If you have sweated a lot during activity, then you will have lost some sodium too. Only when you have replaced this sodium are you fully rehydrated.

Let's say you have lost 2 litres of sweat during activity. You then drink 2 litres of water over the next half an hour. The water is absorbed into the blood, but the blood needs both water and sodium. Just providing water makes the blood dilute. So now we have a situation in which the blood volume is low (dehydration) and the blood is also dilute. To reduce dilution, the body produces urine, which will be clear in color even though you are still dehydrated.

You can increase your sodium levels by doing the following:

- Take a sports drink during and after activity. This will help replace the sodium lost in sweat.
- Eat a meal soon after finishing your activity as the meal will contain sodium. You will still need to drink fluids to replace the fluid lost as sweat.

Taking vitamin supplements is likely to make your pee bright orange all the time as the urine is where a lot of your vitamins end up. In this case you need to drink fluids until you pass copious urine, say, once an hour, to be sure you have enough fluids on board.

Rehydration and Rapid Stomach Emptying

Any fluid you drink needs to pass from the stomach to the small intestine before it can be absorbed and replace sweat losses. Fluid replacement is not a case of how fast you can drink, but of how fast the fluid gets from your mouth and into your blood.

It can take 10 to 20 minutes for fluids to travel from your stomach to your skin for sweating. Sports dietitians recommend drinking fluids early to allow for this delay. People vary greatly in their rates of stomach emptying and intestinal absorption. Factors that may influence stomach emptying include fluid volume, exercise intensity and fluid concentration.

Fluid Volume

Larger volumes will empty from the stomach at a quicker rate. Athletes should begin exercise 'comfortably full' with fluids.

Try drinking 300 to 500 mL (10 to 17 oz) in the 15 minutes before exercise (about two glasses). Then drink around 150 to 250 mL (5 to 8 oz) every 15 minutes during exercise. The idea is to keep a reasonable volume of fluid in your stomach as this improves the rate the fluid empties from the stomach into the intestines and then into your blood. Unfortunately, large

volumes may also increase gastrointestinal distress and the risk of stitch, so you need to get the balance right.

Exercise Intensity

The rate of stomach emptying will decrease in very high intensity exercise, such as sprinting and cycling uphill. It should be noted that not many sports require athletes to maintain that intensity. At a lower intensity, stomach emptying will occur at near-normal rates.

Fluid Concentration

If the sugar content of a drink is too high, the fluid will empty slowly from the stomach. Sports drinks are especially formulated to empty quickly from the stomach. They have a sugar content of 6 to 8 per cent (i.e., 6 to 8 g per 100 mL). Soft drinks (sodas) will have a sugar content of 10 to 14 per cent in most cases, too high for rapid emptying from the stomach. (See chapter 6 for more information on digestion and stomach emptying.)

Sports Drinks

Sports drinks have been around for a while now, with a huge market growth in the 1990s. They were originally based on the theory that because sweat tastes salty, we need a salty drink. That's guesswork, not science. The sports drink has come a long way since then.

There is widespread scientific agreement that sports drinks are of great benefit in replacing both fluid loss and carbohydrate (sugar) burned during sport. Although frequently cited as being most useful during endurance events, sports drinks can also enhance sports performance during intermittent, high-intensity exercise such as occurs in most team sports. Sports drinks also provide sodium to replace the sodium lost in sweat.

Advantages of Sports Drinks

We all know that water is a good fluid replacement drink and is suited to many activities such as walking, gardening and light exercise. We also know that many of us engage in more strenuous and longer exercise, and it is here

Table 5.1 Comparison of the Benefits of Water and Sports Drinks for Fluid Replacement

Benefits of water	Benefits of sports drinks
• Very good for rehydration • Ideal for sports lasting less than 45 minutes • Empties quickly from the stomach and is quickly absorbed into the blood • Cheap and convenient • Good for most children's sports • Does not damage teeth	• Excellent for rehydration • Ideal for sports more than 45 minutes • Helps avoid hyponatremia in ultra-endurance events • Empties quickly from the stomach and is quickly absorbed into the blood • Low cost, especially if made from a powder • Good for teenage and adult high-intensity or endurance sport • Acidic so should be swallowed without washing around the mouth (water is better as a mouth rinse) • Taste preferred by most athletes, therefore often consumed in larger amounts than is water

that the sports drink comes into its own. This section details the advantages a sports drink can offer the athlete, with a summary of the benefits of water and sports drinks listed in table 5.1.

Carbohydrate

The carbohydrate in sports drinks, mainly in the form of the sugars glucose and sucrose, delays fatigue by topping up blood glucose levels to provide glucose for the active muscles. It may also spare muscle and liver glycogen stores, which is very important in exercise exceeding 90 minutes. Research at the University of Iowa in the United States suggests that sports drinks with two types of sugar stimulate significantly greater water absorption than those with only one type of sugar.

Most sports drinks are 6 to 8 per cent carbohydrate (i.e., 6 to 8 g of carbohydrate in every 100 mL). It was once thought that a drink that was more than 2.5 per cent carbohydrate slowed the rate at which fluids left the stomach. Additionally, researchers believed that glucose polymers (chains of glucose molecules, sometimes called maltodextrins) were more suited to sports drinks as they emptied from the stomach faster. The range of sugars normally found in sports drinks is shown in figure 5.5.

More recent research has revealed that a drink with up to 8 per cent carbohydrate will

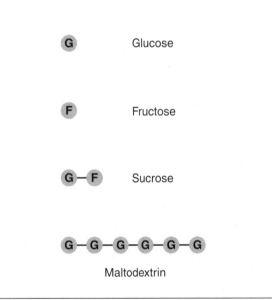

Figure 5.5 The different kinds of sugars found in sports drinks.

empty quickly from the stomach and it doesn't really matter what form the carbohydrate takes, although the glucose polymer is less sweet so may be better suited to some people's taste. Once the carbohydrate level is higher than 8 per cent, fluids will empty more slowly from the stomach, which means that water is available to the body at a slower rate. During sport, avoid drinks that are over 8 per cent carbohydrate. See table 5.2 on page 81 for a comparison of fluid replacement drinks.

A sports drink should be used to provide 30 to 60 grams of carbohydrate per hour of endurance exercise as that is the common rate at which carbohydrate is burned during exercise. Half a litre (17 oz) of sports drink will provide around 30 grams of carbohydrate.

Concentration

Most sports drinks are labeled as 'isotonic', which means that the fluid has a similar concentration as blood. Isotonic fluids quickly empty from the stomach into the small intestine where they can be rapidly absorbed into the bloodstream.

Hypertonic fluids are more concentrated than blood and cause water to move from the blood back into the intestine to dilute the fluid. This effectively causes a transient dehydration before the fluid can be absorbed. Generally, drinks with more than 8 per cent carbohydrate (e.g., regular soft drinks, fruit juice and energy drinks) will be hypertonic.

A *hypotonic* fluid has a lower concentration than blood. Water is a common example, and some sports drinks are slightly hypotonic. Hypotonic and isotonic solutions are absorbed more quickly than are hypertonic solutions.

Salt (Sodium)

Salt (or sodium) is added to sports drinks not just to replace the salt lost in sweat but also to enhance the fluid absorption from the intestines, although carbohydrate concentration may be a more important influence on absorption. Some drinks include magnesium, which doesn't seem to improve absorption or assist sports performance.

Added sodium also improves the taste of sports drinks, which generally contain 250 to 500 mg (11.0 to 21.5 mmol/L) of sodium per litre. This is a higher level than found in tap water, and similar to that found in milk.

The more important benefit from the sodium in sports drinks is in helping to maintain plasma volume. In the recovery period after exercise, full rehydration doesn't occur until all sodium losses have been replaced. The sodium in sports drinks helps the body retain ingested fluids rather than just 'renting' them.

Fit people generally have a higher blood volume than those who are sedentary. Taking a sodium-containing drink before exercise can further increase blood volume, leading to an improvement in endurance.

If, during ultra-endurance sports, sweat losses are replaced solely by a low-sodium beverage such as water, the athlete may suffer from hyponatremia (low blood sodium). All ultra-endurance athletes should include a sports drink with sodium to avoid this condition.

After sport, fluids need to be replaced in greater amounts than sweat loss as some fluid will be converted to urine even if the body is still dehydrated. Without sodium, much of the ingested fluid will pass via the urine.

Protein?

Early evidence suggests that a drink with both protein and carbohydrate can benefit athletes. Protein may reduce muscle damage during exercise and enhance the replacement of glycogen stores after exercise. One study (Saunders, Kane and Todd 2004) showed that endurance cyclists were able to ride for 29 per cent longer when their sports drink contained 1.8 per cent protein (1.8 g per 100 mL). What must be remembered is that this research was on well-trained cyclists who rode to exhaustion. The effect may not be the same for recreational athletes who train and play for fitness and enjoyment.

Sports drinks with added protein are currently on the market. Further research will clarify whether they consistently benefit athletes, and if they do, whether only elite athletes gain that benefit, or anyone doing an hour or more of exercise each day. It's just too early yet. That is the nature of science—information and research is gathered from many sources before clear guidelines can be given.

Other Considerations for Your Sports Drink

Although the carbohydrate concentration and sodium levels are very important aspects to the value of a sports drink, further considerations influence the enjoyment and suitability of your sports drink choice.

Drink Temperature

It's best to keep your drink cool unless you are competing in very cold conditions. If you can't refrigerate your drink, then freeze it so it has just thawed by the time you get to drink it. The drink temperature doesn't appear to affect the speed at which the drink empties from the stomach and is absorbed by the intestines. If you exercise in cold temperatures, you may prefer a drink at a warmer temperature.

Taste

Research using athletes shows they will generally drink more of a flavoured drink than just plain water both during exercise and after exercise. This holds true for children, adolescents and adults alike. So if you are at risk of dehydration because of the intensity of exercise, the air temperature or the length of the event, you will be better off with a flavoured drink that you enjoy. (Note: The flavour you enjoy when rested may be different to what you enjoy when you are exercising, so choose your favourite flavour when you are hot and sweaty.)

Carbonation

I do not recommend carbonated (fizzy) drinks during sport. Fizzy drinks are absorbed at a much slower rate than noncarbonated drinks, such as water and sports drinks. One research group found that fizzy drinks empty from the stomach three times slower than flat drinks. Fizzy drinks are also difficult to drink quickly and give you the burps.

Who Should Take a Sports Drink?

Now that you have seen the potential benefits of a sports drink to athletes, let's take a look at which athletes would benefit most under different circumstances.

- **Recreational athletes.** The sugars in sports drinks can be useful in continuous aerobic activity longer than 90 minutes (if glycogen stores are well stocked before exercise). The sports drink may have value in shorter events if you haven't eaten enough carbohydrate before the event.

- **Elite athletes.** If you are an elite athlete, you may train for two or three hours, or have two or more training sessions in a day. A sports drink will be handy to get you through the demands of training.

- **Endurance athletes.** Because of your very high kilojoule needs, you will need a sports drink throughout long training sessions and endurance events. A sports drink will help maintain normal blood glucose levels near the end of endurance events or long training sessions. Sports drinks also improve sprint times at the end of an endurance session. This can be particularly important in some events. For example, many long-distance cycle events end with a sprint to the finish. Start drinking early to get the most benefit.

- **High-intensity training athletes.** When the sessions are fast and furious, glucose and glycogen are burned at a faster rate and may run out after 30 to 45 minutes of sprint training. A sports drink will let you train for longer. Drink as often as possible throughout training.

- **Tired athletes.** The most common cause of tiredness in athletes is not eating enough carbohydrate. Check that you are eating enough carbohydrate before and after training. A sports drink will help provide additional carbohydrate during sport.

- **Recovering athletes.** If the session has been long and exhausting, then a sports drink can help you rehydrate and restock your glycogen stores quickly. It's great for endurance and elite athletes who must replace lost fluids and carbohydrate quickly, especially if the next event or training session is less than eight hours away.

- **Athletes who don't like water.** Athletes generally prefer a flavoured drink over plain water both during and after exercise.

- **Athletes exercising in the heat.** Glycogen is burned up at a faster rate during exercise in the heat, possibly as a result of an overheated cardiovascular system unable to provide enough oxygen and fat to the muscles.

- **Cramping athletes.** Some athletes lose a large volume of sweat during their sport. The sodium losses can accumulate over a couple of hours, and the resulting low blood sodium will initiate cramps. Some athletes have very high sweat sodium levels, making them even more prone to cramping. The sodium in a sports drink helps replace lost sweat sodium (see the section on stitches and cramps at the end of the chapter).

- **Thin athletes.** If you find yourself losing too much weight during a season, then the carbohydrate in a sports drink may reduce your body's desire to use up your fat and muscle as fuel.

Which Sports Drink Is for You?

Choose a sports drink that suits your taste and budget, and has no more than 8 grams of carbohydrate in 100 mL. Under warm to hot conditions, it must also be one you can drink 800 mL (27 oz) or more of in an hour. If you sweat a lot, I suggest one with more than 15 mmol/L of sodium. For economic reasons, I also suggest you buy the powdered version of sports drinks. Cordial and fruit juice may be diluted 50:50 and used as a sports drink if you wish, but they will be low in sodium and are not ideal for the serious adult athlete. Table 5.2 shows a comparison of the various drinks on the market and indicates which of the sports drinks are most suited to sport based on our criteria for carbohydrate and sodium.

Other Types of Drinks

Apart from water and sports drinks, other drinks are popular with athletes, with some not delivering all the benefits they might imply. None are harmful in sensible amounts, but they each have some angle you will need to consider.

Energy Drinks

A number of so-called 'energy' drinks are on the market. These are not sports drinks and are not recommended before, during or after sport. Many will contain caffeine (often in the form of guarana) and have a sugar content similar to that of soft drinks (10 to 13 per cent) so they will be absorbed more slowly than a sports drink will. Most provide 40 to 80 milligrams of caffeine in a 250 mL (8 oz) can—the equivalent to a cup of coffee or two cups of tea. This can be a shock to those who don't drink other caffeinated beverages, although the caffeine in one can will be well handled by regular tea or coffee drinkers. Please remember that these are not sports drinks.

Sports Waters

Since the birth of the sports drink and the energy drink, there has emerged the sports water. As a general rule, they are low in carbohydrate and sodium; hence, they are not a true sports drink. Enjoy them, but as refreshment, not as a fluid replacement drink during training or competition.

Alcohol

Most elite athletes now give alcohol a miss during their sport season. Some coaches have a 'No alcohol' policy during the season, whereas others prefer a more lenient 'No alcohol in the 48 hours before competition' policy. Most high-level coaches I know will also have a 'No alcohol if injured' policy. In 1990 Australian Commonwealth Games swim coach Don Talbot placed an alcohol ban on all swimmers, coaches and officials throughout the Auckland Games. Despite the myth, alcohol is not sweated out. Only 2 per cent of alcohol appears in the sweat; over 90 per cent of it is metabolised by the liver, which can be destroyed by too much alcohol. So can the brain. That's why alcohol needs to be respected.

You have heard that alcohol can be good for your health. Sensible amounts appear to reduce the risk of heart disease and possibly dementia. One or two standard drinks (10 to 20 g alcohol) maximum each day can provide some health benefits, but more than that is linked to increased risk of stroke and liver and

Watch Those Fangs

Any fluid with a pH below 5.5 has the potential to damage the enamel on the outside of your teeth. The pH is a measure of acidity of food and drink. Examples of fluids with a low pH are fruit juice, soft drinks (regular and diet), wine, beer and sports drinks. The latter has been targeted as a cause of tooth enamel erosion, especially in young athletes (Milosevic 1997). This is unfair, as most people drink far more fruit juice and soft drinks than they do sports drinks. If you drink lots of juice, soft drinks, cordials or sports drinks, please see your dentist every six months.

Although sports drinks have a low pH, the pH on the surface of the tooth returns above pH 5.5 within five minutes as a result of the buffering action of saliva, thereby halting enamel erosion (Millward et al. 1997). To minimise any tooth enamel erosion, follow these guidelines when drinking juice, soft drinks or sports drinks:

- Drink cold fluids (cold reduces acidity).
- Don't swish fluids around the mouth; swallow them quickly.
- Drink by the mouthful rather than constantly sipping small volumes.

Table 5.2   Comparison of Fluid Replacement Drinks

Drink	Carbohydrate (g) per serve	Carbohydrate per 100 mL	Sodium (mmol/L)	Caffeine (mg)
Sports drinks				
Gatorade, 250 mL (8 oz)	15.0	6	21	0
Powerade, 250 mL	20.0	8	11	0
Adams Ale Sport, 250 mL	15.0	6	10	0
Staminade Sport, 250 mL	17.0	6.8	12	0
Hyposport, 250 mL	16.8	6.7	24.6	0
pb sports, 250 mL	17.0	6.8	25	0
Lucozade Sport, 250 mL	16.0	6.4	21.7	0
Sports waters				
Powerade light, 250 mL	6.7	2.7	11	0
Powerade sports water, 250 mL	6.2	2.5	5.2	0
Mizone sports water, 250 mL	6.2	2.5	0.5	0
Waterplus (Sanitarium), 250 mL	0	0	2.6	0
Thorpedo, 250 mL	11	4.5	11	0
Energy drinks				
Red Bull, 250 mL	28	11.2	34	80
V, 250 mL	28	11.2	47	50
Lift Plus, 250 mL	31.5	12.6	8.6	36
Black Stallion, 250 mL	27	10.8	20	80
Waters				
Water, mineral water, soda water	0	0	Variable	0
Soft drink and cordials				
Soft drinks, av., 375 mL (13 oz)	45	12	6.5	0
Cola soft drinks, regular, 375 mL	40	11	5	50
Diet soft drinks, 375 mL	0	0	5	0
Diet cola soft drinks, av., 375 mL	0	0	5	50
Flavoured mineral water, 375 mL	40	11	7	0
Cordial, 250 mL	25	10	7	0
Lucozade energy, 300 mL (10 oz)	52	17	10	0
Juices				
Fruit juice, av., 250 mL	25	10	2	0
Fruit juice drinks, av., 250 mL	25	10	2	0
Tomato juice, av., 250 mL	10	4	40	0

Note: Some drinks in this table have different volumes.

Table 5.3　Standard Drinks and Alcohol Units

Standard drinks	
Drink	**One standard drink (approx.)**
Low-alcohol beer (2–3% alcohol)	570 mL (1 pint [UK]; 20 oz)
Regular beer (4–5% alcohol)	285 mL (half pint [UK]; 10 oz)
Wine (12% alcohol)	100 mL (3 oz)
Fortified wine (e.g., port, sherry; 20% alcohol)	60 mL (2 oz)
Spirits (e.g., whisky, gin, rum; 40% alcohol)	30 mL (1 oz)
Alcohol units (UK)	
Drink	**One alcohol unit (approx.)**
Low-alcohol beer (2–3% alcohol)	1 pint
Regular beer (4–5% alcohol)	half pint
Wine (10% alcohol)	100 mL (3.4 oz)
Fortified wine (e.g., port, sherry; 20% alcohol)	50 mL (1.7 oz)
Spirits (e.g., whisky, gin, rum; 40% alcohol)	25 mL (0.8 oz)

brain damage. See table 5.3 for standard drinks and alcohol units. In Australia, the National Health and Medical Research Council (2003; p. 165) stated that the long-term risk associated with alcohol rose when men consumed five or more standard drinks a day and when women consumed three or more standard drinks a day. Lower amounts are recommended to women because they metabolise alcohol more slowly and have a smaller body mass than men do. Note that beer is around 3 mmol/L sodium—far less than the recommended 15 to 20 mmol/L in today's sports drinks.

During competition I myself once received incalculable help from beer. The race was the 1977 Thanksgiving Day 25 km Turkey Trot in Poughkeepsie, New York. I had been pursuing a runner for 10 or 12 miles and, unable to gain a yard, had despaired of catching him. Without warning he stepped off the road, rummaged in a pile of leaves, withdrew a can of beer he had apparently secreted there earlier, popped open the top, and stood drinking it as I passed. I never saw him again until he came across the finish line a minute or more after I had arrived.

James Fixx, The Second Book of Running, 1978

Following are five reasons to respect alcohol:

• **It is dehydrating.** Alcohol has a dehydrating effect on the body. It reduces the ability of antidiuretic hormone (ADH), the hormone that regulates urine production. As the name implies, this hormone stops you from producing too much urine. With ADH out of action, you can drink six glasses of wine but pass a greater volume of pee. Smart athletes don't drink alcohol in the 48 hours before an event, nor straight after the event until they are well hydrated. Beer with an alcohol content less than 2 per cent doesn't seem to act as a diuretic. I suggest that you fully rehydrate before you drink any alcohol, but a light beer or two later probably won't be of any harm.

• **It slows injury recovery.** Alcohol increases the diameter of blood vessels to the skin, arms and legs (hence the red eyes and flushed face). The increased blood supply will make any injury bleed and swell more than normal. Conversely, an ice bag, compression and elevation of the injured part will reduce swelling and bleeding. Smart athletes don't drink alcohol in the 24 hours after injury.

• **It is fattening.** Although it is not as fattening as fat and fatty foods, alcohol still has the ability to make you gain extra body fat. Excess alcohol is also often associated with a greater consumption of greasy snack foods, chips and take-aways. Smart athletes drink only sensible amounts of alcohol so they stay in control of their eating.

- **It weakens your thinking.** Alcohol can encourage you to do some silly things and stops you from thinking smart. It can also distract you from eating and drinking for optimal recovery after training, when you need to rehydrate and replace your glycogen stores before the next workout. Alcohol also slows the rate of glycogen replacement after sport, giving you a longer recovery time.

- **It is not a good source of carbohydrate.** Beer has a reputation for being a high-carbohydrate drink. This is not true. One can of beer (375 mL [13 oz]) provides around 10 grams of carbohydrate. As a pre-event meal you would need 10 to 20 cans to get enough carbohydrate. Those left standing shouldn't present too much of a problem to the opposition.

Tea, Coffee and Cola

It is often said that caffeine-containing drinks are diuretics and, like alcohol, should be avoided before and after sport. There is little evidence to back this view. All three drinks are good sources of fluids. This is backed by a statement from the Institute of Medicine (11 February 2004), which said the following: 'While concerns have been raised that caffeine has a diuretic effect, available evidence indicates that this effect may be transient, and there is no convincing evidence that caffeine leads to cumulative total body water deficits. Therefore, the panel concluded that when it comes to meeting daily hydration needs, caffeinated beverages can contribute as much as noncaffeinated options'. However, as mentioned in this chapter, these drinks aren't the best choices during sport or immediately after. Cola and other fizzy drinks should not be consumed during sport, but once you have rehydrated, they can be refreshing and contribute to your fluid needs. Tea, coffee and colas shouldn't be discounted simply because of their caffeine content, but they aren't the optimal fluids to use before, during or after exercise as the rate of absorption of fluid into the body will not be as fast as that of sports drinks or water. See the section on caffeine in chapter 8 for more information.

Cramps

We have all experienced that excruciating knot of painful involuntary muscle spasm that can stop us dead in our tracks. About two out of three athletes have experienced the cramp. It commonly occurs in the calf, thigh or foot.

What triggers a cramp? Nobody knows for sure. Surprisingly, this topic is poorly covered in most sports medicine books. Cramps tend to occur more frequently with age. There have been some anecdotal reports that creatine supplements may cause cramps. It is suspected that the most common causes in athletes are dehydration, overexertion or a poor blood supply to the muscle. Heavy sweat losses can cause significant salt (sodium) losses from the body, and this can trigger a cramp if the sodium isn't replaced. Elite athletes commonly lose a lot of sweat and sodium. To combat the threat of cramp, they add some extra salt to their meals and take a sports drink throughout training and competition. A study of a tennis player who regularly got cramps revealed that he lost more sodium through sweat than he ate in his diet (Bergeron 1996). By taking a sports drink and increasing the sodium in his diet, he was able to reduce the cramps to rare occurrences.

In 2002, I was fortunate to accompany Brett Lee, Australian fast bowler, to the Gatorade Sports Science Institute in Chicago, USA. In the laboratory Brett was subjected to sweat sodium measurements. His sweat was quite high in sodium, around 1,300 milligrams per litre, and those losses became a potential problem over a six-hour day of fielding and sweating in which he may lose 6 litres or more of sweat. Brett often suffered cramps in the last hour of play, but since he started taking a sodium supplement (Gatorlytes), the cramping hasn't returned.

The following is the best advice for avoiding cramps:

- Drink plenty of fluids to avoid dehydration.

- If you lose a lot of sweat during exercise, especially over an hour or more, drink a sports drink to help replace the lost sodium. The meal following exercise will also help replace sodium losses.

- Be fit. Cramps are less common in athletes who are well trained.

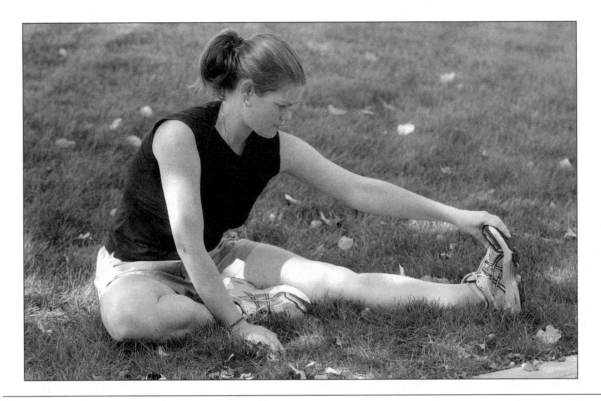

Figure 5.6   To relax a calf muscle that is cramping, grab the toes and ball of your foot and pull them toward the kneecap.

- Eat well. Cut the fat that clogs arteries. Cramps occur in muscles that have a reduced blood supply as a result of narrowed arteries.
- Stretch before and after exercise. If you suffer night cramps, stretch before going to bed.
- Wear proper clothing. Loose, comfortable clothes are best. Tight-fitting clothes can reduce blood flow to muscles, making them more susceptible to cramps.
- Acclimatise to the warmer weather to help avoid dehydration.

If you do get a cramp, stretching the cramped muscle is the best way to reduce the pain. If it happens in the calf, grab the toes and ball of your foot and pull them toward the kneecap, as shown in figure 5.6. This helps the muscle to relax. Applying ice can also stop the spasm and reduce the pain.

The Stitch

As with the cramp, very little research has been done on the stitch, yet so many of us have suffered sharp pain in the abdominal region at some stage during exercise. The stitch is now referred to as exercise-related transient abdominal pain (ETAP). The stitch occurs most commonly in the midabdominal region and, strangely, more often on the right side than on the left. Younger people are more prone to the stitch, and fitness provides some protection against it. However, the stitch still occurs in many fit people. Different sports have different rates of the stitch. One study showed that each year about 70 per cent of runners and swimmers experienced the stitch, whereas the stitch occurred in only one third of cyclists and about half of basketballers and aerobics participants.

It is unclear as to what exactly is 'the stitch'. One theory is that blood flow to the diaphragm drops and the lack of blood causes pain. Another theory is that the pain emanates from stress on the ligaments from the diaphragm to organs in the abdomen as a result of the jolting motion of sport, but that can't explain why swimmers get the stitch. The third theory, and the one that best fits the symptoms, suggests that stitch pain is due to the two membranes of the parietal peritoneum rubbing together and causing a friction pain (see figure 5.7). The outer layer attaches to the abdominal wall, and the

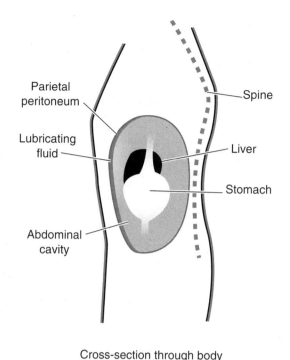

Cross-section through body

Figure 5.7 It is believed that the two membranes of the parietal peritoneum rubbing together generate the pain experienced as the stitch.

inner layer covers the organs inside the abdomen (stomach, liver, spleen). Between the two layers is lubricating fluid, so that the two layers can move across each other during any movement of the torso. The parietal peritoneum can get irritated from the following:

- Dehydration reducing the fluid level between the two membranes, promoting friction
- Distention of the stomach pushing the two membranes together

- Increased movement in the abdominal region during some sports

Based on the preceding, the best advice for avoiding the stitch is as follows:

- Don't eat in the two or three hours before sport. This will allow ample time for the stomach contents to empty into the small intestine.
- Don't become dehydrated.
- Drink small amounts of fluid frequently during exercise. This will help avoid stomach distention and large volumes of fluid bouncing around inside the stomach.
- Drink only water or sports drinks as these empty more quickly from the stomach than other fluids do.

Here are other tips that work for some people:

- Bend forward and push on the affected area.
- Breathe out with pursed lips.
- Wear a wide cloth belt (like a cummerbund) that can be attached firmly around the waist.

Have you ever had a 'shoulder stitch'? If you have, you know exactly what I mean. If you haven't, then, like me, you'll be thinking, How can you have a shoulder stitch? Well, it seems that parts of the parietal peritoneum are linked to the phrenic nerve. When the parietal peritoneum experiences pain, it 'refers' the pain up to the shoulder. Weird, isn't it?

FINAL SCORE

- It's easy to lose 1 litre or more of sweat during each hour of exercise. Sweating is a very good cooling mechanism. Try to replace sweat losses during sport.
- Grab that drink. Don't wait until you're thirsty. Thirst is not a good indicator of fluid needs during exercise. Drink before, during and after exercise. Be well hydrated before you start exercising.

  Before: 300 to 500 mL (two to three glasses) in the 15 minutes before exercise

  During: 150 to 250 mL (5 to 8 oz) every 15 minutes

  After: Replace all lost fluids (you'll probably need at least 500 mL [17 oz])

- Practice drinking at training. In warm weather, aim to be able to drink 800 mL (27 oz) or more each hour. Don't miss an opportunity to drink. Don't wait until you are thirsty. Thirst during sport means you are very dehydrated.

(continued)

- After sport, rehydrate *before* drinking alcohol. Water is a good choice. Athletes with high energy needs may choose sports drinks, fruit juice, cordials or soft drinks. Drink nonalcoholic fluids until you are properly hydrated before you consider drinking any alcohol.
- Drink fluids until you pass clear urine. If you take vitamin supplements, your urine is likely to be a darker colour anyway. In that case, drink until you pass copious urine frequently.
- For more information on fluids in sport, download the free fact sheets #1 and #19 from www.sportsdietitians.com.

part II

Practical Food Choices for Training and Competition

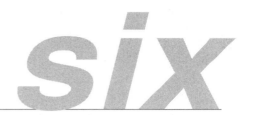

Digestion and Timing of Meals

Way back in 1822, French Canadian Alexis St. Martin accidentally received a gunshot wound to the stomach. Fortunately, U.S. Army surgeon William Beaumont was able to save his life, although on healing there remained a hole in St. Martin's abdomen through which Beaumont could place his fingers and see inside his stomach! For the next few years Beaumont did a series of 238 'physiological experiments' in which food was introduced through the opening and observed for the rate of disappearance and production of hydrochloric acid by the stomach. Beaumont discovered that all foods and all combinations of food were digested. He wrote his findings in 'Experiments and Observations on the Gastric Juice and the Physiology of Digestion', published in 1833.

St. Martin said that he went through a lot of pain to teach the world about digestion. I'm sure that you too have gone through some pain learning about your digestive system. Have you ever suffered nervous diarrhea right before a big competition, or been slowed down by the pain of heartburn during exercise? They can be just as debilitating as the cramp or stitch discussed in the previous chapter. In this chapter we take a look at the digestive system, where food and drink are broken down into small molecules that are then absorbed into the blood. We will travel through the digestive tract and see what happens to our meals as they go from mouth to south. Along the way, I will tackle some myths of digestion. I will also look at how our knowledge of the digestive system is relevant to active people. By the end of the chapter, you'll have a good idea of what happens to your food once you eat it and how you can control some of the most common gastrointestinal upsets.

Stage 1: The Mouth

Chewing is a very important part of your enjoyment of food. Although most of your taste buds are on your tongue, saliva is necessary for experiencing the flavours from food (try dabbing your tongue dry with a paper towelette and sprinkling some sugar on your tongue—you can feel something there but you can't taste the sugar until you mix it with saliva). Saliva also lubricates food to facilitate swallowing, and it starts carbohydrate digestion through an enzyme called amylase.

Finally, saliva plays an important role in protecting your teeth from decay. When a food is eaten and some carbohydrate remains in the mouth, oral bacteria feed on the carbohydrate and produce lactic acid. This acid can break down tooth enamel and begin the process of decay. Saliva then comes to the rescue. The minerals in saliva (calcium, fluoride and phosphorus) help remineralise teeth after each snack or meal as long as at least two hours pass between meals or snacks. Naturally, brushing your teeth regularly also helps. Athletes who are constantly dehydrated may not produce enough saliva to keep their teeth healthy. This is a good reason to keep well hydrated during and between sporting events.

Stage 2: The Stomach

Once chewed and mixed with saliva, the food goes down the throat and lands inside the stomach. The stomach plays the role of a food warehouse with a capacity of around 1,000 to 1,200 mL in adults. Only a small amount of digestion happens here, and no nutrients are absorbed from the stomach. The two main functions of the stomach are as follows:

- To add hydrochloric acid to the food, with the aim to kill some of the nasty bacteria you may have eaten
- To liquefy everything you have eaten, as the small intestine (it follows the stomach) can deal only with liquids

The stomach does secrete a little protease enzyme to help kick-start protein digestion, but this is only a minor function. The majority of digestion doesn't occur in the stomach, but in the small intestine.

Now, you might think the food inside your stomach is inside your body. This is not so. The lining of your digestive tract is just an extension of your skin; the cells of the skin 'specialise' to become lips, tongue, throat, stomach and intestinal lining before exiting via the anus to return to being normal skin again (see figure 6.1). In a fashion, you are like a giant doughnut; the hole in the middle is your digestive system. Whatever is 'inside' your stomach and

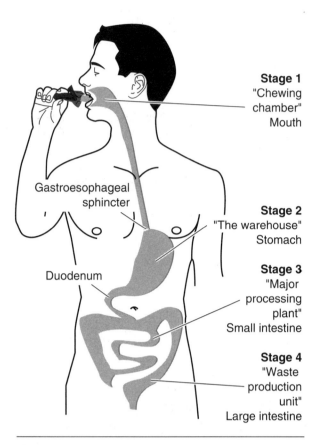

Figure 6.1 The digestive system comprises four main stages, with each playing an important role in processing food.

intestines is still really 'outside' your body. Not until the food has been digested and absorbed into the blood is it technically inside the body. This mainly happens in the small intestine, the next stage. The importance of this concept will become evident soon.

A low-fat meal will empty from the stomach faster than a high-fat meal will—in fact, usually within two hours. That's why a fatty meal can make you feel sluggish—it can take three or four hours to exit the stomach. Sports dietitians suggest that athletes eat a high-carbohydrate, low-fat meal two to three hours before exercise or training, to allow time for it to empty from the stomach. This is especially important in running-based sports in which comfort depends on an empty tummy.

Drinking water with meals will also help your stomach to empty faster. It is a misconception that drinking water with meals slows down the rate of digestion. Food that has been diluted by water with a meal will empty more quickly into the small intestine. In addition, the digestive enzymes can work more efficiently on diluted food.

Can You Eat Protein and Carbohydrate Together?

You may have heard that you should not eat high-protein and high-carbohydrate foods in the same meal because some claim that protein and carbohydrate together won't digest and will ferment in the stomach. There is no scientific evidence for this. It is perfectly OK to eat protein and carbohydrate, or meat and vegetables, together. Your digestive system has the capacity to digest and absorb nutrients no matter the combination of foods or when you eat them. William Beaumont's experiments on poor Alexis taught us that over 170 years ago. And since 1935 we have known that the pancreatic enzymes for the digestion of protein and carbohydrate are secreted simultaneously regardless of the type of food eaten. Why do people say that protein and carbohydrate eaten together won't digest and will ferment in the stomach? I'm not sure, but they are way, way, way out of date, and there isn't a dietitian in the world who will back that claim.

Of course, if you couldn't digest protein and carbohydrate together, then most of the world's population would be in trouble. The most popular food on the planet is rice, a delicious combination of protein and carbohydrate. Likewise for bread, pasta, legumes, milk, yogurt and many vegetables. Breast milk is the perfect blend of protein and carbohydrate, along with some fat. Women don't have one breast labeled protein and the other, carbohydrate! And don't believe the old story about meat taking six weeks to digest. Meat generally requires about four hours to be fully digested in the small intestine.

During sport, fluids in the form of water or sports drinks will empty the most quickly from the stomach, as explained in the previous chapter. As fluids cannot be absorbed from the stomach, they must move from the stomach to the small intestine as quickly as possible. It is here that all liquids are absorbed to replace sweat losses.

Stage 3: The Small Intestine

When the stomach contents have been liquefied, the liquid from the stomach then trickles into the first part of the small intestine at around one or two teaspoons per minute. Most of the digestion and absorption of food and water happens in the 6.5 metres (21 ft) of the small intestine, especially in the first part called the duodenum (see figure 6.1 on page 90). The process of digesting a meal in the small intestine will generally take about two hours. (This is in addition to the two to three hours it can take to empty from the stomach.)

As shown in figure 6.2, during digestion, protein is broken down to short chains of

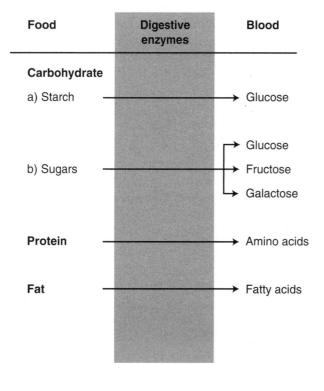

Figure 6.2 The process of digestion breaks down large molecules found in food to smaller components to be absorbed into the blood to nourish the body.

amino acids, fat is broken down to fatty acids, and carbohydrate (sugar and starch) is broken down to its sugars, primarily glucose and fructose.

Now that the food is broken down into smaller molecules, it can be absorbed into the blood, where it is officially 'inside' your body. This concept is important to remember when you are taking fluids. Concentrated fluids such as soft drinks take some time to empty from the stomach and be absorbed from the intestine, whereas sports drinks and water will be absorbed much more quickly.

Because of the natural delay between the time fluid enters the stomach to the time it is absorbed from the intestine, I tell athletes to start drinking fluids *before* they begin training or competition. With 250 mL (8 oz) of fluid taking about 20 minutes to empty from the stomach, this delay before absorption needs to be considered. Drinking early means that fluids are being absorbed around the same time fluid is being lost as sweat. Waiting until, say, 30 minutes into sport until you drink means that your body may not start replacing sweat until the 50-minute mark, and in that 20 minutes you may have lost another 300 mL (10 oz) of sweat.

If food is too concentrated for the small intestine to deal with immediately, it requests water to dilute the contents. There are two ways this happens. Either you drink more water with your meals, or the intestines take some water from your blood temporarily to perform the dilution. The first way is smart. The second way creates mild dehydration, which is not a problem if you are just watching TV. It could be mildly problematic, however, if you are going to train in the following two or three hours.

If your exercise is of a lower intensity, say, walking or recovery training, then digestion and absorption will continue during exercise. It will stop only during intense exercise, which may only be occasional in your sport (e.g., short sprints in netball or football). If your sport involves sprint work or high-intensity work such as circuit training or hill climbing, then you will definitely need an empty stomach, or the contents may revisit your mouth and burn your throat. Virtually everyone has experienced heartburn (a misnomer as it is your throat that is burning), and it is extremely common in running-based sports. Undigested food that has mixed with hydrochloric acid in the stomach is forced up through the gastro-

esophageal sphincter and into the throat. The stomach is designed to accommodate acid; the throat isn't.

Generally, your aim is to get food from the stomach to the small intestine as soon as possible so that nutrients and fluids can be absorbed to fuel active muscles and replace fluids lost during sweating. That is, only when food and fluid have moved from within the tube inside your body to within your blood can we say it is truly 'inside your body'.

Stage 4: The Large Intestine

The remaining bits and pieces of your meal (mainly fibre and a little starch and protein that is resistant to digestion) move past the appendix and enter the large intestine, so called because it has a wider diameter than the small intestine. Here, water absorption is completed and healthy bacteria have a feast on the fibre and leftovers to produce protective compounds against bowel cancer.

The waste spends about 18 to 30 hours in the large intestine if you have chosen a healthy diet with adequate fibre (much longer if you haven't eaten enough fruit, vegetables and whole-grain cereal foods). If the diet contains plenty of fibre, the bacteria proliferate to make the waste soft and bulky and easy to pass. The normal range for bowel motions is once every three days to twice a day. Once a day may not be normal for everyone.

The Quickest Way From the Stomach to the Small Intestine

It is not comfortable to have food in your stomach before competition or training. So how do you get valuable nutrients quickly from your stomach into your small intestine to be digested and absorbed and into your blood? Consider the factors shown in figure 6.3 and expanded on here.

1. **Avoid concentrated foods.** Foods with a high kilojoule concentration such as high-fat foods or high-sugar drinks will empty slowly from the stomach. Avoid soft drinks just before, or during, sport as they are very concentrated and empty slowly from the stomach. The fluids

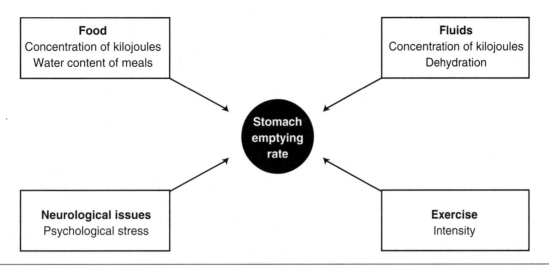

Figure 6.3 Factors that affect stomach emptying.

that empty the most quickly from the stomach are water and sports drinks. A meal of fish and chips could take four to five hours to empty from the stomach, whereas a meal of steamed rice, stir-fried vegetables and lean meat may take only two hours to empty. It's best to eat high-carbohydrate meals with little fat as they will empty from the stomach in about two hours. Low-fat snacks such as a banana or low-fat yogurt empty in about an hour or so. Drinking some water with meals will help dilute the kilojoules and allow quicker emptying from the stomach.

2. **Consider liquid foods.** Liquids will empty from the stomach more quickly than solids will. Sometimes athletes prefer not to have solid foods before sport because it makes them feel uncomfortable, so a liquid meal such as a smoothie, Sustagen Sport, low-fat flavoured milk or a low-fat soy beverage is ideal.

3. **Keep topping up.** The more fluid you have in your stomach, the faster it will empty into the small intestine for absorption. When drinking fluids during exercise, don't let fluid empty completely from the stomach before you have another drink, if possible. Keep topping up with fluids every 10 to 15 minutes.

4. **Don't dry out.** Dehydration during exercise will slow stomach emptying. This can be a problem for the athlete trying to replace lost fluids as quickly as possible. This is the reason athletes are told to start drinking very early in exercise, well before they are thirsty or have a dry mouth.

5. **Relax.** When you are hurried and anxious, food will empty more slowly from the stomach. Sometimes a bit of anxiety can't be helped, especially before important events, job interviews and exams. If you are the nervous type, allow a little more time between the pre-event meal and the event, say, three to four hours. (Unfortunately, anxiety can have the opposite effect on the large intestine, giving you the squirts. If you get turbulent insides during sport, see the following section.) Physical pain can also slow down stomach emptying.

6. **Consider your exercise intensity.** The stomach will empty normally during low-intensity exercise (e.g., walking, jogging), but as the intensity increases, the emptying rate will slow down. This rarely presents a problem as high-intensity exercise is not maintained for long periods. Games that involve intermittent high-intensity exercise (e.g., soccer, basketball) can cause a slight reduction in the stomach emptying rate.

Note: There is some evidence that women have a slower stomach-emptying rate than men and therefore may be more prone to heartburn. There is also a great deal of variation among people in their stomach-emptying rate; what works for you may not work for others.

Gastrointestinal Upsets: Solid, Liquid or Gas?

It's happened to just about all of us. There we are, deep into a training session, and our insides start playing a strange symphony. It's usually athletes involved in running-based or endurance sports who suffer the problems of tummy upsets, wind and diarrhea. Such conditions are also more common during high-intensity exercise and as the training schedule becomes longer and harder. Let's examine some common problems and potential solutions.

Urgency

The need to have a bowel movement in the middle of training or competition can be quite distressing. It's also quite common. Some people even have to arrange their training so it's close to a toilet.

The urge is more likely to occur if exercising just before the normal time of toileting. It occurs most in running-based sports, possibly because the constant pounding of feet on the ground quickly pushes waste through the descending colon of the large intestine.

Possible Solutions

• If possible, train yourself to have a bowel movement before exercise. Conversely, schedule training after you would normally have a bowel movement.

• Warm liquids can have a gentle laxative effect. A hot cup of coffee or tea before an event can stimulate the movement of waste through the large bowel.

Stomach Cramps, Intestinal Cramps, Abdominal Bloating, Diarrhea

About half of all triathletes and long-distance runners suffer some kind of intestinal trouble in events and training. Swimmers, rowers and cyclists are less likely to experience such trouble, probably because they are in weight-supported sports and don't jangle their insides around as much as those in running-based sports do.

There isn't a simple answer that will solve everyone's problems. If none of the following suggested remedies solve the problem, or if you see blood in your stools or vomit, see your sports physician immediately.

Possible Solutions

• Avoid highly concentrated drinks and supplements. Some high-kilojoule drinks and supplements such as amino acids are very concentrated and will drag water from your blood into the bowel, giving cramps, bloating and possibly loose stools.

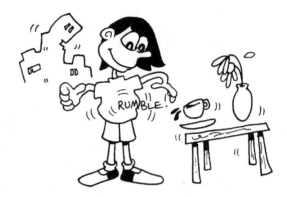

• Eat two hours before sport. People who vomit or get stomach cramps during exercise are likely to have eaten too close to training or the event.

• Drink plenty of fluids. Gut problems are more common in people who are dehydrated. Blood flow to the intestines is reduced in exercise by 70 to 80 per cent. This is normal. But when an athlete is dehydrated, this blood flow is further reduced, possibly causing a disturbance in the normal function. Drinking water or sports drinks is unlikely to be a cause of stomach cramps, unless large volumes are drunk at once.

• Beware of fructose. Fructose is a sugar appearing in most carbohydrate foods, notably fruit and fruit juices. The intestines have a limit as to how much fructose they can absorb. If too much fructose is eaten in one hit, some ends up in the large intestine where resident bacteria use it to produce substances that cause diarrhea. Large amounts of fructose can be taken by drinking lots of apple juice, grape juice and the juices in many canned fruits. Eating four to six pieces of fruit a day is unlikely to cause fructose problems.

Nervous Diarrhea

Almost everyone has experienced the need to have a bowel movement just before an event. The long queues at the toilet before the start gun are testimony that many people experience this reaction. The cause is probably anxiety and stress.

Possible Solutions

• There is no simple solution. If you can find a way to relax, you may just solve this problem.

• Take a spare toilet roll to events, just in case the public toilets become unreliable.

• Remember that diarrhea can have a number of causes such as food poisoning or celiac disease.

- If diarrhea persists beyond the pre-event time, please see your physician.

Nausea and Vomiting

Nausea and vomiting occur more frequently in athletes who eat close to the event (less than one hour), have too much fat in their pre-event meal, or have taken highly concentrated fluids such as soft drinks or energy drinks just before sport. In all cases the food or drink has taken longer to empty from the stomach, and some contents still remain in the stomach.

Possible Solutions

- Eat two hours before sport. Make sure the meal is low in fat and high in carbohydrate.

- Try liquid meals. They tend to empty more quickly from the stomach and will minimise problems with nausea or vomiting.

- Avoid highly concentrated foods such as fatty foods and regular soft drinks.

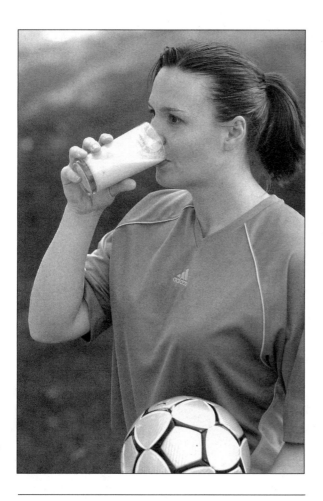

Liquid meals will empty more quickly from the stomach than solid food will. This can be advantageous to the athlete who gets nervous before sport or is pressed for time.

Heartburn

Heartburn is caused by food being in the stomach at the time of exercise. The acidic contents of the stomach come up past the gastroesophageal sphincter and into the throat, giving a burning sensation.

Possible Solution

Ensure that the stomach is empty before you start exercise or sport. You can usually avoid heartburn by eating a high-carbohydrate, low-fat meal at least two hours before the event.

Endurance Diarrhea

Stomach cramps, diarrhea and sometimes fecal incontinence can occur near the end of a marathon or triathlon. During intense exercise, blood supply to the intestines is reduced. If exercise continues for a long time, and dehydration occurs, the intestines can lose control over their contents.

Possible Solution

Drink sufficient fluid to avoid dehydration. Diarrhea during endurance sport is much more likely to happen if you are dehydrated. Keep those fluids up!

Burping

Burping is not usually a hazard on its own, just more of a nuisance. It commonly occurs when drinking fizzy drinks or eating food so quickly that lots of air is swallowed with the food. The gases accumulate in the stomach, to be released later as a burp.

Possible Solutions

- Choose nonfizzy drinks such as water and sports drinks.

- Eat and drink slowly in a relaxed setting to avoid swallowing air with food and drink.

Flatulence

A bit of wind is quite normal but can become an ill wind that blows no good if abdominal cramps are also present. It is caused by gas being pushed through the last part of the colon.

Possible Solution

Avoid wind generators such as cabbage, Brussels sprouts and legumes (baked beans, kidney beans) in the two meals before the event.

Constipation

Constipation is uncommon in athletes as moderate exercise is usually very good for getting waste to move efficiently through the digestive system. Constipation may occur during travel across time zones or between countries, or if you are forced to change from your regular diet.

Possible Solution

Choosing higher-fibre versions of carbohydrate foods (whole-meal breads, fresh fruits, baked beans, vegetables) will definitely help relieve constipation. If constipation is caused by travel, you can expect your bowel habits to return to normal after about 48 hours.

Possible solutions for gastrointestinal problems are summarized in table 6.1. You may need to experiment to find the solution that works best for you.

Table 6.1   Summary of Gastrointestinal Problems in Athletes

Problem	Possible solution
Urgency	Have a bowel movement before exercise.
Stomach cramps, bloating, diarrhea	Eat at least two hours before exercise. Avoid dehydration. Avoid concentrated drinks such as soft drinks and fruit juice.
Nervous diarrhea	Try relaxation methods.
Nausea and vomiting	Start exercise with an empty stomach. Avoid concentrated drinks such as soft drinks and fruit juice.
Heartburn	Start exercise with an empty stomach.
Endurance diarrhea	Avoid dehydration during the event.
Burping	Eat slowly and avoid fizzy drinks.
Flatulence	Avoid 'windy' foods.
Constipation	Eat higher fibre foods.

FINAL SCORE

- The main function of the digestive system is to break down the large molecules in your food into small molecules that can be absorbed into the body.
- Protein is broken down into amino acids.
- Carbohydrate is broken down into sugars, mainly glucose.
- Fat is broken down into fatty acids.
- Athletes generally need to allow a couple of hours for the stomach to empty before they engage in sport and should be familiar with the factors that influence stomach emptying.
- If food remains in the stomach while exercising, athletes have a much higher risk of heartburn, nausea and possibly vomiting.
- Many gastrointestinal upsets can be prevented by following the simple solutions presented in this chapter.

seven

What to Eat Before, During and After Exercise

> I came out with high energy, which I have been lacking in the last couple of games. I think it was the baked beans on toast for pre-game.
>
> *Basketballer Lauren Jackson during the women's world basketball championships (2002)*

Dietary advice to athletes has changed over the years. In the beginning it was purely speculation and experimentation, before science gave us a better understanding. We now know that what you eat, and when you eat it, will make a big difference to how you perform.

Nutrition Before the Event

Some people eat far too close to an event or training session and find themselves feeling quite unwell soon after the start of exercise. I met a footballer who wouldn't eat after his 8:00 a.m. game-day breakfast because he thought he might vomit during the game. His problem was that he was hungry and tired by game time. 'Any ideas?' he asked. Well, as the game didn't start until 3:00 p.m., I introduced him to the concept of lunch. He thought that the stomach took over a day to empty.

Some of the concepts mentioned in chapter 6 on digestion are relevant when discussing the best food and fluids to consume around sport. The following sections address key issues regarding eating before exercise.

High Carbohydrate and Low Fat

The preexercise meal needs to be high in carbohydrate to top up your glycogen stores for endurance. The glycemic index (GI) of the foods will probably have little bearing on your performance unless that performance is longer than 120 minutes, but you might want to experiment with the low GI foods as described in chapter 3. For a guide to how much carbohydrate you need just before, during and just after exercise, take a look at table 7.1. For example, a light meal of 75 to 150 grams of carbohydrate will suit most people (about 1 to 2 grams per kilogram of body weight) as a preexercise meal. The same amount of carbohydrate will be needed after exercise to start the process of replenishing muscle glycogen stores. After a moderate amount of exercise, say, a 60- to 90-minute workout, you will need 5 to 7 grams of carbohydrate per kilogram of body weight in the following 24 hours, which is 350 to 490 grams for a 70-kilogram (154-lb) person.

Table 7.1 Approximate Carbohydrate Needs for Sport

Timing	Carbohydrate intake
Before exercise	1–2 g per kg body weight about 2–3 hr before exercise
During exercise	30–60 g per hr of endurance exercise (e.g., 500–1000 mL [17–34 oz]) sports drink per hour
After exercise	1.0 g per kg body weight soon after exercise finishes 5–7 g per kg body weight during 24 hr after moderate exercise 7–12 g per kg body weight during the 24 hr after heavy exercise

Note: Women may require the lower end of the carbohydrate range given.

The preexercise meal should also be low in fat so that it empties as quickly as possible from the stomach and into the small intestine where it will be digested and absorbed into the blood. Food remaining in the stomach when you begin your activity is likely to make you feel uncomfortable, especially in running-based sports, because the food can 'joggle' up and down inside the stomach. Remember, only absorbed food can fuel the body. See chapter 3 for examples of high-carbohydrate, low-fat eating.

Moderate Protein

Some people will tell you that you should eat plenty of protein before a workout or a hard training session. Unfortunately, there is no evidence to back that claim. Of course, there is a very good chance that your preexercise meal will contain a reasonable amount of protein anyway as it is likely to include milk, cereal, bread, pasta, rice, meat or fish.

You may prefer a food bar as part of your pre-event meal, and most of these will contain some protein. As long as you are eating enough protein over the day, your body and muscles will be happy. See chapter 2 for more information on protein.

Table 7.2 provides some ideas for meals and snacks that are high in carbohydrate, low in fat and varying in protein.

Timing of Meals and Snacks

Two to three hours is usually enough time for the stomach to empty before the event. Most low-fat, light meals will empty from the stomach within two hours. Almost all meals will be out of the stomach within three to four hours.

How close you eat to an event is up to you, but consider the following:

- You generally need to allow more time for running-based sports, such as football, netball and hockey, as any food remaining in the stomach will bounce around and make you feel uncomfortable. The food may also rise through the sphincter at the top of the stomach and burn the lining of the throat (heartburn).

- You can eat closer to the event in sports in which your body weight is supported, such as swimming, rowing and cycling. Put another way, weight-supported sports may be performed with a small amount of food in the stomach and not upset the athlete.

- Any sport that involves physical contact to the stomach such as boxing, rugby or wrestling will require an empty stomach to help you avoid embarrassing moments.

- Allow more than three hours between meals and sport if you get nervous. Anxiety will slow the rate at which the stomach empties. This is usually an important consideration before important sports events.

- Liquid meals, such as fruit smoothies and low-fat flavoured milk, tend to empty more quickly than solid foods. This is a very efficient way to get food into your body if you don't want solid foods or you get nervous before events.

- Sometimes it isn't convenient to eat a couple of hours before exercise, such as when you have an early morning training session. In that case, ensure that your meal and snacks before you go to bed are high in carbohydrate. Consider diluted fruit juice or a sports drink on waking before a long early morning training session. These will top up your glycogen stores before you start.

Table 7.2   High-Carbohydrate Meals and Snacks

Meal or snack	Protein (g)	Fat (g)	Carbohydrate (g)
1 medium baked potato 1/2 cup baked beans 1/2 cup mushrooms	9	1	30
200 mL (7 oz) low-fat yogurt 1 Tbsp dried fruit	10	1	35
Fruit smoothie (made of 200 mL nonfat milk + banana)	10	0	35
1 cup breakfast cereal 150 mL (5 oz) low-fat milk 1/2 cup canned fruit	11	1	55
2 slices raisin bread 2 Tbsp ricotta cheese 1 Tbsp jam	7	5	45
45 g (1.6 oz) lean ham and salad 1 bread roll 1 fresh fruit	15	3	45
1 cup spaghetti or baked beans 2 slices toast	12	3	60
2 cups breakfast cereal 200 mL (7 oz) low-fat milk 1/2 cup canned fruit	17	2	90
2 slices toast 1 Tbsp honey 240 mL (8 oz) fruit juice	6	2	65
1-1/2 cups steamed rice 1-1/2 cups stir-fried vegetables 100 g (3.5 oz) lean meat	35	6	90

Sugar Before Sport

Many claim that eating sugar, or a sugar-containing food, before sport can ruin your performance. The premise is that the sugar causes high blood glucose levels, which causes high levels of insulin to be released into the blood, resulting in low blood glucose levels and poor performance. This assumption is based on one study published in 1979. Although this study showed a reduction in performance after eating carbohydrate in the hour before sport, most subsequent studies have shown either a neutral effect or a performance boost of 7 to 20 per cent. It's interesting that these haven't received as much publicity as the study over two decades ago. (You will recall that a sharp rise in blood glucose levels probably doesn't occur, as sugar, or sucrose, has a moderate glycemic index.) A glass of soft drink (250 mL [8 oz]), for example, has a moderate glycemic load of 14.

So, don't take the old truism as natural law. Experiment with foods and fluids and find out what feels best for you. If you believe sugar is a 'downer', then avoid it; if you think it's your 'upper', then please enjoy a small sugar boost. It's your body.

Carbohydrate Gels

Conveniently packaged, and popular with runners and triathletes, is the carbohydrate gel (e.g., Carboshotz). A 50-gram sachet provides 34 grams of glucose. Many athletes will slip these inside their shorts and retrieve them when required. As they are a concentrated source of carbohydrate, I strongly suggest you experiment with them during training. Although

Lack of Appetite Before Sport

Even if you aren't hungry, it is still smart to eat some form of carbohydrate food, especially if you are endurance training or playing sport in the morning after a sleep. If you don't fancy a solid meal, think liquid. A smoothie (see recipes in chapter 11), fruit juice or other commercial low-fat liquid meals are good choices. Low-fat liquid foods will generally empty from the stomach within two hours.

Special Foods

As yet, there is no particular food that can be taken just before sport to improve your performance. But many athletes truly believe that a specific food makes a big difference. If you believe a certain food helps your performance, then eat it. It's called the placebo effect. A footballer once told me that he always eats bananas before a game because the first time he had a pregame banana he was judged 'best on ground'. Just as the cricketer puts the left pad on first for good luck, you should choose whatever food or drink you think is lucky for you.

Relaxation

A lot of people get nervous before big events. Relaxing can be a difficult task for many athletes concerned about an impending event. Some will feel nauseated; others will suffer loose bowels or frequent urination. If you get tummy trouble, read chapter 6 for advice. Anxiety can slow the rate of stomach emptying, so you may benefit from taking a liquid meal.

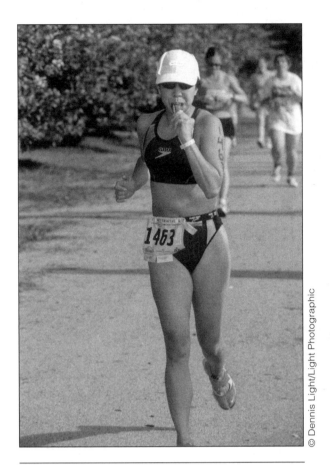

© Dennis Light/Light Photographic

Carbohydrate gels can be a boost to the endurance athlete.

they can be consumed on their own, it makes physiological sense to dilute them by washing them down with water (around 400 to 500 mL [14 to 17 oz] for every 30 grams of carbohydrate). The dilution will encourage the glucose gel to leave the stomach and enter the intestine more quickly than if it were just eaten alone. As a guide, have one 50-gram sachet in the 10 minutes before the start of an event, and then one or two 50-gram sachets per hour of sport.

Burger Power

It was Mike's first world record to be set without eating a McDonald's hamburger and fries before competition.

News sheet from the U.S. team when U.S. breaststroker Mike Barrowman broke the 200-metre world record at the 1992 Barcelona Olympics. It was the sixth time he had broken the world record since 1988.

There isn't a sports dietitian in the world who would recommend a burger and chips before the big event, but it goes to show that not everyone listens, and yet some can still perform well despite our advice. Let's be fair—he was in the water less than two minutes, not a time span that would sap his glycogen stores. I'm willing to bet his usual pre-event meal would not have helped him in the 1,500-metre event.

Fluids

Avoiding dehydration is crucial to your performance. You should be well hydrated before you start an event. I suggest you drink an extra 300 to 500 mL (10 to 17 oz) in the 15 minutes before you start, even if you don't feel thirsty. Why this can be a distinct advantage is covered in chapter 5 on fluids. Water is an excellent sports drink. Use a commercial sports drink if you don't fancy water, if the session is of high intensity, or if the event is likely to last more than an hour.

Nutrition During the Event

There is no doubt that you need fluids during exercise. Try to drink around 150 to 250 mL (5 to 8 oz) every 15 minutes during exercise, the bigger amount in warm weather. Don't wait until you are thirsty. If you feel thirsty, you are too dehydrated to perform at your best.

If you've read this far, you know that carbohydrate is important at every stage of the athlete's diet. Scientists aren't certain how carbohydrate consumed during an event may improve endurance, but it's probably due to the following:

- Sparing muscle glycogen. In low-intensity exercise carbohydrate taken during the event can be remade into glycogen for later use.

- Sparing liver glycogen. The extra glucose taken orally means that the liver doesn't have to produce as much glucose to maintain blood glucose levels.

- Keeping blood glucose (sugar) levels normal during moderate- to high-intensity exercise and providing extra fuel for empty muscles.

Near the end of an endurance event, blood glucose levels will gradually drop and could get low, making you feel faint or tired. Consuming carbohydrate during sport will keep blood glucose levels up, providing glucose for muscle energy, and therefore delaying fatigue. Of course, you will feel tired eventually during sport depending on your training and muscle glycogen stores before the event. Guidelines for eating and drinking vary depending on the type of event.

Team Sports and Shorter Events

Most team sports and individual events are completed within 90 minutes of action (e.g., netball, squash, football, soccer, field hockey or a 10-km [6-mile] jog). There is no advantage in eating solid foods during these sports as there wouldn't be enough time to digest and absorb the food. Besides, solid food will probably feel uncomfortable in your stomach. If you feel tired during the event, then you probably didn't eat enough carbohydrate before the event, you are undertrained or you are overtrained.

Fluids are very important in all exercise, and should be taken during these sports. To replace glycogen stores and blood glucose, many athletes eat jelly beans or other soft confectionery at the half-time break of many sports. They will need to be washed down with water to assist absorption. It can be helpful to take a sports drink to provide some carbohydrate and help delay fatigue in a short event, but proper nutrition before the event is the best move to avoid fatigue during sport.

Endurance Events

Events over 90 minutes long are generally considered endurance events. You can go along easily for 90 minutes if you were well fuelled before you started. Unfortunately, because we don't have a never-ending supply of glycogen fuel, in endurance events an athlete should try taking more carbohydrate fuel on board while on the move, like a jet fighter taking a mid-air refuel.

The carbohydrate found in a sports drink will help delay fatigue. If you eat solid food, then it should be one you know will not upset your digestive system. For example, jelly beans, jelly snakes, muesli bars (low fat, of course) and bananas are popular solid foods with long-distance athletes.

Experimentation on athletes shows that around 30 to 60 grams of carbohydrate per hour should be consumed in an endurance event to delay fatigue (the lower amount for smaller athletes, or lower-intensity exercise). This is the equivalent to 500 to 1,000 mL (17 to 34 oz) of sports drink or 10 to 20 jelly beans.

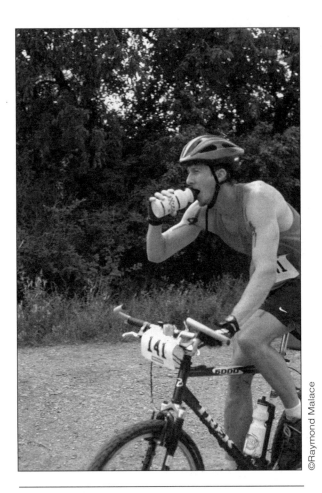

©Raymond Malace

Taking a sports drink during exercise provides valuable carbohydrate and fluids.

Ultra-Endurance Events

For events over four hours, the ultra-endurance athlete trains and competes at a lower intensity than that of short-distance events and most team games. As exercise intensity at less than 70 per cent maximum heart rate may not interfere with digestion, the athlete could consume high-carbohydrate foods with small amounts of protein and fat such as muesli bars, breakfast bars, jam sandwiches and hot soups (if the event is held in cold conditions). Ultra-endurance athletes may find foods with a higher glycemic index preferable because of their more rapid digestion.

Liquid meals are popular with ultra-marathoners. If this is your sport, try commercial food drinks such as Sustagen Sport during training to see whether they agree with your constitution.

Ultra-endurance athletes should enlist the help of an experienced sports dietitian because of their very high energy and nutrition requirements. Many will need over 21,000 kilojoules (5,000 cal) a day just to maintain their body weight and get the energy they need each day. Ultra-marathoners who completed a 100-kilometre run consumed an average of 4,200 kilojoules (1,000 calories) with a range of 1,970 to 8,000 kilojoules (470 to 1,920 cal) during the run. Their favourite solid foods were potatoes and bananas, and their favourite drinks were sports drink, water and soft drinks (Fallon et al. 1998).

When glycogen stores get low, the body begins to use protein as a muscle fuel. Even if glycogen stores are reasonable, a small amount of protein is used as a fuel source near the end of endurance events. This implies that endurance athletes need more protein. This is true, but see chapter 2 for more details.

Tour de France

Over three weeks, competitors in the Tour de France cover around 4,000 kilometres (2,485 miles), climbing altitudes of up to 2,700 metres. It is considered to be one of the most strenuous sporting events in the world. In fact, during this race one of the highest daily energy expenditures by a human was recorded—a massive 32,700 kilojoules (7,810 cal).

Researchers from the University of Limburg, The Netherlands, found that the cyclists ate an average of 24,280 kilojoules (5,800 cal) and 850 grams of carbohydrate a day. On some days they ate up to 32,400 kilojoules (7,740 cal); that's more than most people eat in three days. Fluid consumption was frequently over 10 litres (2.6 gallons) a day (Saris 1990; Lucia, Earnest and Arribas 2003). Be glad you don't have to pay for their groceries!

World Record a Huge Drag

Tour de France riders have been recorded at over 31.4 megajoules (7,500 cal), and cross-country skiers at 29.3 megajoules (7,000 cal) daily. That was impressive until Mike Stroud from the Institute of Human Nutrition, Southampton, England, and a mate pulled sledges, initially weighing 222 kilograms (488 lb), almost the entire width of Antarctica and through the South Pole (Stroud et al. 1997).

Using the isotope-labeled water technique, their individual daily energy expenditure was measured at a whopping 44.6 megajoules (10,650 cal) and 48.7 megajoules (11,630 cal) during the toughest part of their journey when they had to drag their heavy sledges uphill. During the first 50 days of the trek, the two men burned a daily average of 38.3 megajoules (9,150 calories) and 28.6 megajoules (6,830 calories) each. This dropped down to 26 megajoules (6,200 cal) a day in the latter part of their journey when the sledges were lighter and some of the terrain was downhill.

It's no surprise that the men lost more than 25 per cent of their body weight, despite eating an average of 21.3 megajoules (5,100 cal) a day, 57 per cent of that as fat (330 g fat) and 35 per cent as carbohydrate (around 450 g). Probably the only weight control program that could honestly boast 'All you can eat . . . and still lose weight'. It also demonstrates a rare endurance feat that needed a high fat intake.

The walk had to be abandoned on the 95th day as both men were clearly suffering from severe malnutrition and struggling in high winds and temperatures of −45 °C to −10 °C (−49 °F to 14 °F). The expedition was the first to successfully complete a crossing of Antarctica without the use of aircraft to ferry food and equipment. It was the longest unsupported walk ever made, a distance of 2,300 kilometres (1,429 miles).

Nutrition During Recovery

You may be exhausted and too tired to eat or even think of food after exercise. Or you may have a hunger you could photograph. In both cases your body is crying: Give me carbohydrate and give me fluid! The answer for some athletes is to drive into the nearest take-away or chug down a few beers. Whoops! Fried chicken and fries, or alcohol, are not what your body needs to recover from the exertion of sport. You have exercised for performance, fun and fitness, not to endure 48 hours of feeling tired and lethargic. What you eat and drink can greatly enhance your recovery.

General Principles

After exercise, drink at least the amount of fluid that you have lost as sweat. See chapter 5 for instructions on figuring out the correct amount. You also need to replace your energy stores.

Muscle glycogen can generally be replaced at 5 per cent per hour, so it takes about 20 hours to replace all the glycogen used after a long training session or an endurance event. Generally, carbohydrate is converted to glycogen faster than normal in the two hours straight after exercise because muscles are ready to take up glucose. An enzyme called glycogen synthase is activated with the specific job of making more glycogen, and muscle cells have an increased ability to absorb glucose from the blood. But, you must remember to eat; without carbohydrate, glycogen replacement is very slow.

Take advantage of this increased speed of glycogen replacement. Eat food and fluids high in carbohydrate. Try to eat 50 to 100 grams of carbohydrate in the two hours after exhausting exercise. You may prefer to take in carbohydrate in liquid form such as fruit juice, soft drinks, sports drinks, commercial meal replacement drinks or your own liquid concoction such as a smoothie. The bonus here is that the fluids you are taking with your carbohydrate are also replacing fluids lost through perspiration. To recover quickly, you will need to drink nonalcoholic fluids until you pass clear urine.

You may choose high glycemic index foods, but if you have at least 24 hours before the next training session, it probably won't matter what form of carbohydrate you choose, just as long as you eat enough of it. Eat enough carbohydrate and you will refill your muscle glycogen fuel tank within 24 hours. (The GI is covered in more detail in chapter 3.)

Although some have suggested that eating some protein with the carbohydrate after exercise quickens the remaking of muscle glycogen, this process seems far more dependent on carbohydrate than on protein. One study showed that consuming a liquid supplement providing about 50 grams of protein and 160 grams of carbohydrate (half straight after finishing exercise and half two hours after exercise) resulted in one and a half times more glycogen being stored (Zawadski, Yaspelkis and Ivy 1992). Other studies indicated that if athletes eat enough carbohydrate after sport, glycogen will be replaced quickly. If athletes eat only a small amount of carbohydrate with protein, the protein seems to enhance glycogen stores more than expected (Burke, Collier and Beasley 1995).

Be aware that there is a good chance that you will eat both protein and carbohydrate together in the next meal after sport. High-carbohydrate foods such as bread, rice, potatoes, pasta, breakfast cereals and food bars contain protein, and you might combine them with high-protein foods such as milk, yogurt, meat, eggs or fish. Recreational athletes training one hour a day may not benefit from adding protein to their postexercise meals; however, further research may show that elite athletes who train twice or more a day will benefit from a posttraining supplement that offers both carbohydrate and protein.

Multiple Events

If you are competing more than twice in one day or competing two or more days in succession, how well you eat will make a huge difference to recovery and performance in subsequent events. The common question is this: What do I eat between events? Following is a simple guide to food and drink choices. Choose one or more items to match your appetite, your sport and the time you have before the next event. For example, if you have 90 minutes before the next event, you might choose a sports drink, a handful of jelly beans and a banana. If you have two and a half hours before you are active again, a sandwich or a tub of yogurt, with a piece of fruit, a cup of coffee and a bottle of water could be ideal.

Less Than One Hour Between Events

Try a combination of one or more of the following:

- Water (provides fluid only)
- Sports drink (fluid and carbohydrate)
- Soft confectionery such as jelly beans (carbohydrate)
- One small banana (carbohydrate)

One to Two Hours Between Events

Try a combination of one or more of the following:

- Water (provides fluid only)
- Sports drink (fluid and carbohydrate)
- Fruit juice, fruit juice drinks (fluid and carbohydrate)
- Soft drink (fluid and carbohydrate)
- Smoothie (fluid, carbohydrate and protein)

Tired?

Not surprising if you have had a hard training session or completed a tough event. How quickly you recover depends on your choice of food and drink. Skimping on carbohydrate is the most common nutritional cause of tiredness in athletes. See the Fatigue Guide (table 4.3) in chapter 4 for causes and remedies of tiredness.

- Piece of fruit such as a banana or apple (carbohydrate)
- Soft confectionery such as jelly beans (carbohydrate)
- Liquid meals (fluid, carbohydrate and protein)

Whatever you choose, don't overfill yourself, or you may feel sluggish for the next event. Fluids will exit more quickly from the stomach than solid foods will. If your events are short (e.g., swimming 50 to 400 metres), then you might find you need only water or a sports drink between events.

Two to Three Hours Between Events

In this situation you have more time to relax and digest your chosen meal. If you are really hungry, consider a banana sandwich; pasta, rice or potato salad; a muesli bar; a breakfast bar; a fruit bar; and other low-fat, high-carbohydrate snacks such as canned or fresh fruit. Use the Nutrient Food Value Chart on page 171 as a guide.

Again, don't overeat, and make sure you have fully replaced your fluid losses from the previous event. (This is a good reason to weight yourself before and after events; the weight lost is mainly in the form of sweat.) Your fluid replacement can include tea and coffee, as well as other nonalcoholic drinks. The meal should be small and provide mainly carbohydrate, protein and fluid, and be low in fat for quick digestion. This is not the time to eat large meals or fatty take-aways. As always, you know your body best, so try some ideas of your own.

More Than Three Hours Between Events

The eating advice for meals between events that are more than three hours apart is similar to that offered in the section on pre-event eating earlier in this chapter:

- Replace all your fluid losses.
- Eat to replace the muscle and liver glycogen used during the previous event.

FINAL SCORE

- Meals in the 48 hours before sport should be high in carbohydrate and low in fat so the meal is digested quickly and maximises muscle glycogen stores. Aim for 1 to 2 grams of carbohydrate per kilogram of body weight in your presport meal.
- Sugar-containing food or drinks can be eaten or drunk in the hour before sport. In most cases they will improve performance.
- Fluid is all that is required during most sporting events and training sessions. A sports drink has many advantages in sessions longer than 45 minutes.
- During long events and training sessions, aim to consume 30 to 60 grams of carbohydrate per hour of exercise. Sports drinks are a simple way of achieving this.
- It is important to refuel your body after exercise. High-carbohydrate food and drinks are good choices. Aim for 50 to 100 grams of carbohydrate (around 1 gram of carbohydrate per kilogram of body weight) soon after finishing sport.
- The body relies on adequate carbohydrate intake after sport to quickly replenish glycogen stores. There is some evidence that protein eaten with carbohydrate foods and fluids after sport will enhance glycogen restoration.
- If you are constantly tired, check your carbohydrate intake and make sure you are well hydrated.

eight

Nutritional Supplements

> Iron tablets, wheat germ oils and vitamins are known to be consumed by some young sportsmen and women keen to improve their performances. With the majority of them, there is not the slightest scientific evidence to suggest that they do have beneficial effects. At best, they can be regarded as forms of placebo, with more psychological than physiological benefits.
>
> *Johnny Warren and Andrew Dettre in Soccer in Australia, 1974*
>
> Those athletes who are under particular strain have to drink the fresh blood of soft shelled turtles which I myself have beheaded.
>
> *Ma Junren, Chinese athletics coach, 1993*

The first person to seek a nutritional ergogenic aid could have been Dromeus of Stymphalus, who, in 450 BC, thought that eating muscle could increase his own muscular strength. Aztec warriors ate the hearts of brave foes in the belief that it would add to their own bravery. A crazy idea, maybe, but some of the supplements on the market are based on similar logic. As you can see from the opening quote to this chapter, athletes have been seeking a benefit from supplements for well over thirty years.

Most athletes have experienced fatigue or a performance slump that is difficult to pull out from. If they can't pin down the cause, many consider a nutritional supplement as a possible solution. Other athletes train hard but will search for a supplement to give them the edge over the opposition. If performance improves after taking the supplement, it is easy to assume that the supplement did all the work.

A scientist would now step in and remind us that improvement is not proof that the supplement 'worked'. It may be just a convenient coincidence. Proof only comes when the same result can be repeated time and time again. It's well known that just giving an athlete a pill can improve performance. Belief in the pill can suddenly have a high-octane result. The question remains: What caused the change—the supplement or the psychology? In this chapter, we explore answers to this question. I also identify supplements that have potential benefits, supplements that don't have enough evidence for or against them and supplements that are not recommended.

In the Mind or in the Pill?

Manufacturers of most nutritional supplements tell you how their product *will* improve your performance. As soon as you believe in the supplement, the placebo effect may come into operation as a psychological ergogenic aid, and your performance may improve. Science attempts to separate the true physiological effect of a supplement from the perceived effect. This is best done with the double-blind trial in which athletes are given either the supplement or an inactive placebo that looks and tastes like the supplement. Neither the researcher nor the athletes know what is being taken (hence 'double-blind') until the very end of the trial when an independent person provides the code. If those taking the supplement improve and those taking the placebo do not, then the researchers are onto something big. If both groups improve, then it's likely to be 'in the mind' or just an effect of regular training.

Unfortunately, determining the benefits of nutritional supplements is never as cut and dried as performing a double-blind trial. Scientists can spend years researching the worth of a supplement and still not get an answer. The difficulty comes in trying to measure the benefits. Current equipment may not be sophisticated enough to record a slight improvement in performance. Considering that only a 1 per cent improvement in performance can mean the difference between gold and fifth, it's no surprise that athletes will grab at anything that gives a hint of a performance edge.

Assessing Nutritional Supplements

When assessing the potential value of a nutritional supplement, consider the following:

• Has there been any independent research on the supplement? You will be surprised to find that many supplements have not been researched in healthy athletes.

• If research has been conducted, has it been published in an independent, peer-reviewed, scientific journal? The marketing of some supplements relies on articles written about the product. Articles are not research. Before an article is published in scientific journals, experts in the field review it to make sure it is up to a high standard.

• Is the research relevant to athletes? Many supplements will cite research articles that are unrelated to the claims for the product. One food bar claimed to assist body fat loss, yet none of the research references cited to sup-

port its claim demonstrated any weight loss capabilities.

• Is the supplement patented? If a product has been patented, then the patent holders usually do most of the research because they will directly benefit from future sales. Truly independent research is rarely published in such circumstances.

• Is the majority of research from one researcher or laboratory? The value of a supplement can be determined only if many researchers from different laboratories work independently to assess it under different conditions. This has been done in the case of creatine and sports drinks.

• Has the research been performed on athletes under normal training or competition situations? Just because a product has benefits for people with certain conditions such as heart disease or a nutrition deficiency, it doesn't follow that the same benefits hold for fit athletes.

• Although there may be research suggesting a benefit of a supplement, is there any research showing 'no effect' or possible dangerous side effects of using the supplement? If one research paper shows a positive effect, but 10 others show no effect, then it is disingenuous to mention the positive result and not to say that the balance of evidence is for 'no effect'.

• Is the product suited to your sport? Taking supplemental creatine can benefit sprint and power athletes, but it is unlikely to benefit marathon runners.

• Have other independent scientists, sports dietitians, sports institutes or sports medicine groups offered supporting comments about the supplement?

• Will the supplement benefit you? Research showing a benefit in elite athletes may not be relevant to recreational athletes.

Only when you start asking questions will you be able to determine the value of a supplement. Be aware that many supplement providers will not like your asking questions (because they won't have credible answers) and will rely on the testimonial as 'proof'. If all you get from a supplement company is essentially promotional brochures and personal stories from athletes, then you will know that science has not been able to support the implied benefits of the product. At least your decision to use, or not use, the product will be an informed one.

Frequently, the argument for a supplement is based on flawed logic. A good example of this logic is Royal Jelly. It is assumed that what is good for queen bees is also good for humans. We are told that the queen bee is fed on royal jelly, a mixture of pollen and secretions from the glands of worker bees. This is why she grows to be twice as large as the regular bees and lives for four or five years, compared to 45 days for the worker bees. That is fine for the bee, but who's to say that it's any good for humans?

Based on this logic, we should be eating antelope, as the fastest land animal is the cheetah (96 km/hr), which feeds on antelope. The fastest marine animal is the killer whale (55 km/hr). More plankton for swimmers! Going back to the insect world, it would make far more sense to eat like a flea, which can jump up to 130 times its own height, or dine like a tropical cockroach, which can travel 40 times its body length in one second. Royal Jelly is definitely not recommended for asthma or allergy sufferers as it has triggered fatal asthma attacks.

Testimonials From Famous Athletes

A common, and very powerful, marketing technique is to get endorsement from a famous athlete. Most elite athletes get their talent and prowess from intense training, coupled with healthy eating, positive mental attitude and favourable genes. Because they often train for many hours a day, elite athletes often don't have time to earn money to pay all their training and travel expenses. They are then willing to try supplements and endorse them to earn some cash. It certainly doesn't mean that they have checked the science, if any, behind the product.

Flawed Ingredients Lists

For many supplements, you can never be sure that they contain the ingredients stated, in the amounts stated. More alarmingly, some may have ingredients not declared on the label. This is of great concern to elite athletes who have to undergo drug testing. The World Anti-Doping Agency (WADA) says that around 20 per cent of nutritional supplements have undeclared ingredients that could lead to a positive doping result (WADA 2004). WADA warns that taking a poorly labeled nutritional supplement is not a defence if an elite athlete is asked to attend a doping hearing. Your local sporting authority will provide information on the safest source of a supplement should you decide to take one. In fact, WADA warns,

> Most supplement manufacturers make claims about their products that are not backed by valid scientific research and they rarely advise the consumer about potential adverse effects. The supplement industry is a money-making venture and athletes should get proper help to distinguish marketing strategies from reality.

Current Findings

We will see many sports nutritional supplements more vigorously researched and, no doubt, there will be breakthroughs such as creatine. Most nutritional supplement research has been done on fit young men. The future could see nutritional supplements offering genuine performance benefits to certain subgroups of people, such as young women or the over-55s.

We will now look at some examples of the common supplements on the market, and you

---

Warning: Women and Supplements

Women who are planning a pregnancy, are pregnant or are breast-feeding should not take any nutritional supplement without their doctor's advice. I do not recommend any nutritional supplement (including creatine) to people under 18 years as most have not been tested on their long-term effects on growth and development. Again, seek the advice of your doctor or sports physician, or contact the sports medicine association in your country.

can judge whether they are worth your money. The supplements have been divided into three categories:

- **Those with potential benefits.** These offer benefits to some athletes under certain conditions. (A supplement will rarely benefit every athlete.)
- **Those for which it's too early to tell.** These supplements look promising on the basis of early research, but it is too early to be certain of the benefits, if any, to athletes.
- **Those that are not recommended.** The research for these supplements is either nonexistent or indicates that the supplement has little benefit in sports performance.

Supplements With Potential Benefits

A few supplements can help some athletes, yet not one of them can we say will definitely help you personally. The one exception is the sports drink as every athlete sweats and uses glucose as a fuel. The others discussed here may help you to get a little extra out of your body. You will need to experiment on yourself with an open mind. Naturally, if you exercise purely for health, fitness and pleasure, then good, wholesome eating will provide you with all your body needs.

Antioxidants

Without oxygen you would die. Yet the very oxygen that is keeping you alive is also contributing to your death because oxygen is toxic. Inhaling oxygen naturally produces harmful free radicals as a consequence of normal metabolism. Free radicals are unstable molecules or fragments of molecules that can cause gradual damage to body cells. The free radicals are made much less harmful by antioxidants produced by the body and eaten in the diet.

Exercise can create a 10- to 20-fold increase in oxygen consumption and therefore a subsequent increase in free radical production. It has evoked the idea of the 'oxygen paradox'—that is, exercise (proven to be good for you) increases the level of free radicals (proven to be bad for you).

Does the 'bad' outweigh the 'good'? The answer is no. Research strongly suggests that regular exercisers have a much higher level of their natural antioxidant enzymes to help protect against the free radicals produced in exercise. In addition, regular exercisers eat more food, including fruit and vegetables, which are abundant natural sources of antioxidants, including the vitamins C and E. This has led to the theory that the 'weekend warrior' most requires antioxidant supplements as his or her antioxidant enzyme levels will be lower than someone who exercises regularly throughout the week. It should be noted that regular exercise reduces your risk of bowel cancer, diabetes, heart disease and becoming overweight.

A number of studies have shown a decrease in free radical damage in physically active people who take vitamin E and vitamin C supplements, but contradictory data show no benefit from taking these vitamins as a supplement. Unfortunately, that is the way of science, and it may be another 10 to 20 years before we can fine-tune the message regarding antioxidant supplements in athletes. The message may well be different depending on whether the athlete is strength training, speed training or endurance training. At the moment, some scientists favour the supplement, whereas others see no value in promoting supplements to athletes. Despite the different views, both parties are unanimous in their belief that athletes need to eat plenty of fruits and vegetables to get extra antioxidants.

I don't know of any researcher who has tried to determine the amount of supplement needed, nor do I know of one who has said how much exercise warrants a supplement. As suggested, the regular exerciser is least likely to need a supplement when training, but anyone involved in hard training or competition for 10 hours or more a week should give it some thought. A daily supplement of 10 to 15 milligrams of alpha-tocopherol equivalents (vitamin E) covers the daily intake recommended by most countries and may be a useful adjunct to your normal diet that, for many people, provides only 8 to 10 milligrams daily. Vitamin E appears safe at doses of 200 milligrams or less daily. Vitamin C is abundant in fruits, fruit juice and vegetables, but a supplement of 100 to 200 milligrams daily is unlikely to cause a problem.

Following are some good sources of antioxidants:

- Vitamin E—vegetables, fruits, nuts, vegetable oils, wheat germ, oily fish (such as salmon, mackerel, tuna and herring)
- Vitamin C—fruits, vegetables (such as oranges, Kiwi fruit, strawberries, grapefruit, capsicum (peppers), broccoli, cabbage and peas)
- Carotenoids—yellow-orange fruits and vegetables, dark green vegetables, tomatoes, fruit and vegetable juices

If you prefer to get your antioxidants through good eating, then, as a guide, you will need to eat at least two fruit serves a day (about 300 g [10.5 oz]) and at least 2 to 3 metric cups of vegetables a day (about 400 g [14 oz]). This is not a lot of food and should be a simple task for any healthy, active adult. Unfortunately,

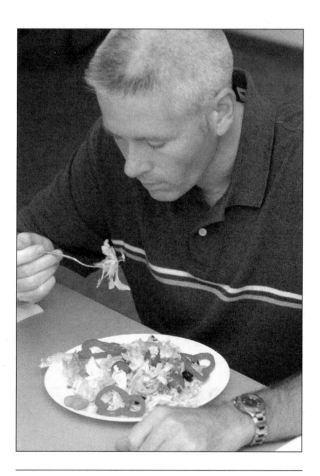

A fresh salad with plenty of vegetables is a good source of antioxidants.

only 1 in 10 adults is eating that much today. Although healthy eating, a supplement or both may reduce oxidative stress, there is no evidence that this will also improve sports performance.

Bicarbonate

During high-intensity anaerobic exercise such as sprinting, lactic acid is produced more quickly than it can be metabolised and can reach a level that causes fatigue. If this lactic acid can be neutralised quickly, then high-intensity exercise can continue for an extended time. Taking a neutralising alkaline salt such as sodium bicarbonate (baking soda) before sprint events has been proposed as an ergogenic aid.

Sodium bicarbonate may be useful in elite athletic events of one to seven minutes' duration, but it doesn't appear to be of any value in events less than 30 seconds or longer than 10 minutes. This is a rare example of a legal, effective and medically safe nutritional ergogenic aid. A typical dose is 300 to 500 milligrams per kilogram of body weight, mixed with water, taken about one or two hours before the event.

Although many studies show the value of sodium bicarbonate supplementation, the effective dose can have a number of unpleasant side effects, such as nausea, vomiting, flatulence, diarrhea and muscle cramps. If the dose is reduced to, say, 200 milligrams per kilogram of body weight, the side effects diminish, but the ergogenic effect is lost too. Drinking plenty of water with the bicarbonate may alleviate the side effects.

Sodium bicarbonate is not banned by the International Olympic Committee, although some say it could be considered in violation of the IOC Doping Rule, which states that athletes shall not use any physiological substance taken in an attempt to artificially enhance sports performance.

Caffeine

Most of our caffeine comes in drinks made from the coffee bean, tea leaf, kola nut and cacao bean in which caffeine occurs naturally (see table 8.1). Plants contain caffeine and related compounds theophylline and theobromine in

Table 8.1　Caffeine Content of Various Foods and Drinks

Drink	Caffeine content
Instant coffee (1 tsp/cup)	60–80 mg/250 mL (8 oz)
Percolated coffee	60–120 mg/250 mL (8 oz)
Drip method coffee	110–150 mg/250 mL (8 oz)
Ground coffee (1 tsp/cup)	25–30 mg/250 mL (8 oz)
Decaffeinated coffee	2–5 mg/250 mL (8 oz)
Coffee substitutes	Caffeine-free
Iced coffee	50–100 mg/300 mL (10 oz)
Tea (1-minute brew)	10–30 mg/250 mL (8 oz)
Tea (5-minute brew)	20–50 mg/250 mL (8 oz)
Tea bag	40–70 mg/250 mL (8 oz)
Green tea	50–80 mg/250 mL (8 oz)
Herbal tea	Caffeine-free
Cocoa	4 mg in 1 tsp
Drinking chocolate	2 mg in 2 tsp
Milo	1 mg in 2 tsp
Aktavite	2 mg in 2 tsp
Ovaltine	negligible
Horlicks	negligible
Guarana powder	76 mg/tsp
Regular cola soft drinks	30–50 mg/375 mL (13 oz)
Jolt Cola	50 mg/375 mL (13 oz)
Diet cola	40–60 mg/375 mL (13 oz)
Caffeine-free cola	negligible
Noncola soft drinks	negligible
Energy drinks 50	50-80 mg/250 mL (8 oz)
Milk chocolate	20 mg/100 g (3.5 oz)
Dark chocolate	60 mg/100 g (3.5 oz)

Note: The large variation in the caffeine content of teas and coffees is due to the variety of beans or leaves, the processing method and infusion times.

their leaves as natural insecticides. Caffeine also appears in guarana and some medications. The chemical name for caffeine is 1,3,7-trimethylxanthine.

Guarana (*Paullinia cupana*) is a Brazilian plant naturally high in caffeine and claimed to reduce stress and depression and increase sports performance. It is a popular soft drink in Brazil, where the guarana paste is mixed with carbonated water and sugar. Any value to athletes is probably more related to its caffeine content. The amount of caffeine present in guarana-containing products is not always stated; therefore, it can be difficult to judge the dose you are taking.

There is so much confusion about caffeine, which is a common ingredient in the Western diet. The brain is the part of the body most sensitive to caffeine. As a stimulant to the central nervous system, caffeine can keep the brain alert. Excessive consumption of caffeine can cause increased urination, nervousness, upset stomach, tremors and irritability. Withdrawal, in those accustomed to high caffeine intakes (500+ mg per day), is associated with headaches, lethargy, irritability and muscle pains, which are usually relieved by a caffeinated drink. Insomnia may occur at 1,000 milligrams a day (about 14 cups of coffee or 8 litres of cola drink).

Is Caffeine a Diuretic?

Technically, caffeine is a diuretic, but that doesn't mean that a cup of coffee will make you urinate excessively. In a review of the literature on caffeine and diuresis, the author concluded that: 'The literature indicates that caffeine consumption stimulates a mild diuresis similar to water, but there is no evidence of a fluid-electrolyte imbalance that is detrimental to exercise performance or health' (Armstrong 2002, p. 201). On averaging the effect of caffeine on diuresis, Dr. Ron Maughan, of Loughborough University, estimated that 1 milligram of caffeine produces 1.17 mL of urine (Maughan 2003). So, if you have a 200 mL (7 oz) cup of tea containing 50 milligrams of caffeine, you will be obligated to produce 60 mL (2 oz) of urine, with the remaining 140 mL (5 oz) being part of your fluid intake.

'Caffeine is a weak diuretic, but this action is often over-emphasised. Recommendations to avoid caffeine use when hydration status may be stressed are probably counter-productive',

said Dr. Maughan. You can see his point: If someone is used to drinking five mugs of coffee a day (about 1,200 mL), that person may not drink the same amount of water if caffeine is eliminated from the diet.

Researchers at the University of Connecticut in the United States tracked 10 athletes for three days while they trained for four hours per day (Fiala, Casa and Roti 2004). The athletes drank water during the training sessions and only cola for the rest of that day, unaware that in one trial the cola had caffeine and in another trial the cola was caffeine-free. Although they drank the equivalent of seven cans of cola drink each day, there was no difference in their hydration levels whether the cola had caffeine or was caffeine-free.

If a caffeinated drink is taken just before sport, or during sport, it won't increase urine production during sport. However, I don't suggest you have caffeine drinks after sport as it may slow the rate at which you rehydrate. Rehydrate with noncaffeine drinks before you enjoy a caffeinated drink.

Caffeine and Sport

Several recent studies show increases in adrenaline levels after caffeine consumption. The extra adrenaline is thought to be useful by improving alertness and reaction times. It may also enhance the use of fat as a fuel and thereby spare glycogen stores. This means that the body should be able to exercise for longer. Not all researchers agree with this theory, as exercise alone makes the body more efficient at using fat. Many athletes find that caffeine reduces the perception of exertion, and this alone might be its greatest effect.

Previously, researchers found that giving endurance athletes doses of 5 to 6 milligrams of caffeine per kilogram of body weight (350 to 420 mg in a 70-kg [154-lb] person) improves performance. The view now is that doses as low as 2 or 3 milligrams per kilogram of body weight (about three cups of coffee in a 70-kg person) provide maximum performance benefits. The consensus is that caffeine has an ergogenic effect in endurance sports, although the best protocol has not been determined. It appears that going 48 hours caffeine-free before taking a 'dose' of caffeine provides the best result.

Caffeine will have different effects on different people. It will depend on how much caffeine is regularly taken during the day, the level of training, the amount of caffeine taken before exercise and genetics. In someone who has very little caffeine normally, two cups of coffee might give such a zing to the brain that it dramatically reduces performance. Someone else may find that exercise is easier and endurance is improved after drinking a caffeinated drink. Some studies show caffeine giving an ergogenic effect in short-duration, high-intensity sports.

The International Olympic Committee (IOC) used to state that the maximum permitted level of caffeine in the urine was 12 milligrams per litre. Above that amount was considered doping and resulted in disqualification of the athlete. In January 2004 caffeine was removed from the list of tested compounds by the World Anti-Doping Agency.

My advice is to give caffeine a try if you wish and gauge your personal performance both with and without caffeine. Try a daily dose of 2 to 3 milligrams per kilogram of body weight—a level now used by endurance athletes and those in team sports. More research on caffeine and the 'dosing' protocol will likely be forthcoming. Whatever you do, experiment during training sessions, not during sporting events. The consensus is that caffeine has an ergogenic effect in endurance sports without any negative effect on hydration.

Carbohydrate Supplements

Supplemental carbohydrate, in the form of powders, gels and sports drinks, can be a very useful adjunct to healthy eating. It will be of most use to athletes involved in high levels of training, endurance sports and high-intensity sports. See chapters 3 and 5 on carbohydrate and fluids.

Creatine

Creatine suddenly became popular after it was claimed that British sprint athletes Linford Christie and Sally Gunnell used it to win gold in the 1992 Olympic Games.

About 95 per cent of creatine is found in skeletal muscle as free creatine and creatine phosphate. You may recall from the first chapter that adenosine triphosphate (ATP) provides the energy for muscle contraction. During intense exercise such as sprinting or weightlifting, ATP will last only one to two seconds.

The role of creatine phosphate is to generate ATP as quickly as it is broken down. There is enough creatine phosphate in muscle to allow ATP regeneration for the first six seconds or so of sprint exercise before glucose can be used to produce ATP. In other words, creatine phosphate helps create enough ATP for the first 50 or 60 metres of a 100-metre running sprint. Thereafter, glucose is broken down to produce ATP for fuel during exercise.

Creatine has a second function of acting as a buffer to reduce lactic acid buildup in the muscle, which further helps to delay fatigue. Exercise increases the creatine content of exercising muscles, so creatine levels are generally higher in fit people.

Creatine occurs naturally in the diet and in the body. It is manufactured by the kidney, liver and pancreas from the amino acids arginine, glycine and methionine. Creatine is found in foods with muscle or nerves (e.g., fish, meat, shellfish and eggs), but we eat only 1 to 3 grams (0.04 to 0.10 oz) of creatine a day through these foods, much less than the experimental amounts used in creatine studies. Unfortunately, cooking tends to destroy creatine. Don't be too concerned if you're vegetarian—although you get less in food, your body will still make creatine.

Fatigue that occurs during very high intensity exercise is associated with the depletion of muscle creatine phosphate. If creatine levels were higher, possibly as a result of supplementation, then creatine phosphate could be remade quickly and plenty would be available for the repeated sprints that occur in sports such as football, rugby, tennis, netball, basketball and soccer.

Research over the last 15 years shows that creatine supplementation improves high-intensity work output probably because the extra creatine accelerates creatine phosphate resynthesis during recovery from intense muscle contraction. In other words, supplemental creatine helps nature restock creatine phosphate stores. Benefits have been shown for repeated sprints up to 1,000 metres.

Creatine should not be viewed as another gimmick supplement; its ingestion is a means of providing immediate, significant performance improvements to athletes involved in explosive sports. In the long run, creatine may also allow athletes to train without fatigue at an intensity higher than that to which they are accustomed. For these reasons alone, creatine supplementation could be viewed as a significant development in sports nutrition.

Paul L. Greenhaff, University Medical School, Queens Medical Centre, UK, 1995 (p. S109)

Recreational athletes will probably see little benefit from taking a costly supplement such as creatine. For the serious amateur and professional athlete whose sport involves sprint work and intense muscle contraction, creatine could offer an advantage.

Despite some claims for banning creatine supplementation, it is not banned by the International Olympic Committee or any other sporting body. There appear to be no harmful side effects when taken in the dose needed for an ergogenic effect. Despite that, creatine supplementation is not recommended for people under 18 years as no one is sure of the effects on growth and development. Neither is anyone too sure of the long-term effects of creatine supplementation.

Creatine Loading

If you haven't taken creatine before, the quickest way to get the maximum levels in your muscles is to creatine-load. Take 5 grams of creatine four to six times a day for a week. Take the creatine with a meal or snack, as carbohydrate (about 70 g) enhances the absorption of creatine as a result of the stimulatory effect of insulin.

This dose seems to increase muscle creatine by about 25 per cent, but it will vary greatly from person to person. You can take a smaller dose (3 to 5 g a day), but it will take longer (about a month) to load the muscles with creatine. When loaded, the muscle creatine content will remain elevated for four to six weeks. To maintain the maximum muscle creatine level, take a maintenance dose of 2 or 3 grams a day. Figure 8.1 illustrates creatine regimens and their corresponding total creatine levels.

Not all athletes will benefit from creatine. Some athletes have naturally high levels in their muscles; others have lower levels. Those with lower levels will benefit the most from supplementation. Lower levels are most likely in vegetarians as they don't eat food with the greatest amount of creatine (meat and fish). (You will only know your creatine levels by having a muscle biopsy, which is impractical for most recreational athletes.)

Creatine seems to work best when there is a short recovery period between sprints, say, between 30 seconds and three minutes, improving performance by 5 to 15 per cent. Creatine is of little value in single sprints such as 100-metre swimming (but it will be useful in training when multiple sprints are required).

There is no evidence that creatine directly increases muscle strength or improves performance in endurance events or low-intensity exercise, although it can increase sprint power during or at the end of an endurance event, such as a cycling race. There is no evidence that

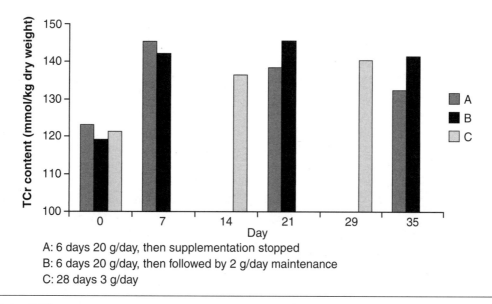

A: 6 days 20 g/day, then supplementation stopped
B: 6 days 20 g/day, then followed by 2 g/day maintenance
C: 28 days 3 g/day

Figure 8.1 Different protocols of creatine loading. TCr = total creatine.

Adapted from E. Hultman, K. Soderlund, J.A. Timmons, G. Cederblad and P.L. Greenhaff, 1996, "Muscle creatine loading in men," *Journal of Applied Physiology* 81(1): 232-237. Used with permission.

creatine provides a useful ergogenic effect for an endurance athlete.

Weight Gain

Creatine supplements may cause an initial weight gain of 1 to 3 kilograms (2 to 6.5 lb) in the first seven to ten days of usage. This is most likely due to water retention, not an increase in muscle size, as some athletes believe. The extra weight may be a disadvantage for sprint athletes (e.g., those in 100 m or 200 m track events), as they will have to transport that weight in their sprints. Over the next couple of months, weight gain may increase to 5 kilograms or more, and this is most likely to be muscle gain due to the extra weight training able to be performed when creatine loaded. The gain in muscle mass is crucial to athletes requiring extra strength in their sport.

Sports Drinks

Sports drinks are designed to replace lost fluids and provide carbohydrate as an energy source during exercise. They are valuable in endurance events and high-intensity exercise. See chapter 5 on fluids for a comprehensive review of sports drinks.

Supplements Without Enough Evidence to Recommend

Some supplements look exciting if you check just some of the research. However, when you look at the balance of all the research, the case for supplementation is less compelling. This doesn't mean that we dismiss the supplement, as the future may unearth some definite benefits. The supplements discussed in this section cannot be widely recommended right now, but further research could see a change in opinion.

Branched-Chain Amino Acids

Leucine, isoleucine and valine are the essential branched-chain amino acids (BCAAs). It has been proposed that BCAAs will reduce mental fatigue in sport, thereby assisting in endurance events. Low levels of BCAAs are associated with higher levels of tryptophan, which in turn is converted to serotonin, a brain neurotransmitter that induces sleepiness. The theory is sound, but the research is less exciting. Some studies show an improvement in sports performance when using 5 to 20 grams of BCAAs daily; others don't.

The BCAAs make up around one third of muscle protein. They are the main amino acids used as muscle fuel near the end of endurance events when glycogen stores are low. Providing extra BCAAs has the potential to improve endurance performance in some people. Indeed, slight improvements in endurance running and cycling have occurred in those taking a BCAA supplement, but these studies have been criticised because they were not well conducted.

The muscle can use leucine for energy, and plasma leucine levels drop during exercise, so it seems logical that athletes may need that additional leucine. A performance advantage for taking supplemental leucine hasn't yet been shown. The overriding message is still to consume adequate carbohydrate to stop muscle protein breakdown.

Glutamine

Glutamine is one of the most abundant amino acids in the body and is made by the muscles, liver, kidneys, heart and lungs. Glutamine supplementation has been proposed for increasing muscle mass and reducing the risk of the flu and other bugs that often afflict the athlete who trains hard or overtrains. As glutamine is involved in muscle synthesis and intense exercise may reduce glutamine levels, it seems plausible that glutamine supplementation will help increase muscle mass. One study revealed that glutamine had a protein-sparing effect at a high dose of 0.9 milligrams per kilogram of body weight, although it didn't influence muscle performance during strength training (Candow et al. 2001). More research is needed before we can recommend glutamine for athletes wanting increased muscle strength and bulk.

Glutamine is an important fuel source for lymphocytes and macrophages, special cells that are part of the immune system. An athlete involved in endurance sports or intense training with little recovery time seems to be more prone to infections, probably because intense exercise puts the body's immune system under stress, causing glutamine levels in the blood to fall. Some research (but not all) suggests that glutamine-supplemented athletes are less likely to get infections. Other researchers see little benefit to glutamine supplements.

Glutamine appears to be safe at daily doses of 0.1 to 0.3 grams per kilogram of body weight.

HMB

Beta-hydroxy-beta-methylbutyrate, or hydroxy methylbutyrate, or just plain HMB, is a popular bodybuilding nutritional supplement introduced to the U.S. market in 1996. It is a metabolite of the branched-chain amino acid leucine and alpha ketoisocaproate, which has also been touted as a bodybuilding aid. The main claims for HMB are that it will increase muscle mass, reduce body fat stores and aid recovery from workouts. The body produces 0.2 to 0.4 grams of HMB each day in the muscle and liver depending on the amount of leucine in the diet, whereas the doses used in research have been 1.5 to 3.0 grams per day. The amount of HMB used in research studies is often more than is found in HMB supplements.

Although a possible action of HMB is not clear, one hypothesis is that HMB inhibits the breakdown of muscle during strenuous exercise, as there are fewer metabolic by-products of exercise-induced muscle damage in the blood and urine following HMB supplementation. If positive effects are eventually proven, bodybuilders, athletes involved in strength training and endurance athletes may see tangible benefits (as they tend to use muscle protein as a fuel source near the end of endurance events).

Professor Melvin Williams, who has over 30 years of research experience with sports ergogenics, has a guarded view of HMB: 'Although the effectiveness of HMB as a sports ergogenic remains to be proven, the preliminary data are somewhat supportive and it appears to be a safe, legal and ethical supplement' (1998, p. 213). More recently, in a review by Steven Nissen at Iowa State University in the United States, the balance of research showed that HMB supplementation of around 3 grams a day enhanced muscle gain and strength when taken in conjunction with a strength training program, doubling the effect of strength training in many cases. This benefit was seen in both men and women, with additional benefits if HMB was taken in combination with creatine (Nissen 2004, p. 163).

Like most sports nutritional supplements, HMB was released onto the market well before its effectiveness could be assessed. Evidence suggests that HMB reduces muscle breakdown and enhances muscle gain. It appears to be safe to use at 3 grams a day. Be warned that there are no studies on the long-term effects of HMB supplementation, and it is expensive.

Supplements Not Recommended

When a supplement has received very little research or the research indicates no benefit to the athlete beyond good nutrition, recommending it to athletes is really unethical. Sadly, many of the nutritional supplements on the market fall into this category. This section looks at a small number of these. Remember that many new supplements arrive on the market each year. I suggest that you follow the guidelines given early in the chapter to assess their value to you.

Amino Acids: Arginine, Lysine and Ornithine

Arginine, lysine and ornithine are amino acids that are often promoted as causing the body to release extra growth hormone, which may then increase muscle growth. An injection of arginine is used to stimulate growth hormone as a test for growth hormone deficiency in children. The injection stimulates growth hormone release for only a short time.

There is no evidence that an oral dose of amino acids stimulates growth hormone release. Even doses of 8,000 milligrams of arginine in an 80-kilogram (176-lb) person haven't been able to stimulate growth hormone release. The average dose of arginine in amino acid tablets is 150 milligrams and in amino acid powders is up to 4,000 milligrams, well below any level that might stimulate growth hormone release.

Ornithine is similar in chemical structure to arginine and lysine, although it is not an amino acid that is used in making body proteins. Injected, ornithine can release growth hormone for an hour or so, but when taken orally in doses up to 10,000 milligrams (10 g) it does not affect growth hormone.

Lysine doesn't appear to increase growth hormone levels in athletes either. Researchers at the University of Helsinki found that giving male weightlifters a total of 2,000 milligrams of lysine, 2,000 milligrams of ornithine and 2,000 milligrams of arginine each day did not change their growth hormone levels (Fogelholm et al. 1993).

In a similar study at the University of Cape Town Medical School, researchers gave 2,400 milligrams of arginine and lysine to body-builders and found no consistent effect on growth hormone release (Lambert et al. 1993). The researchers summarised that there 'is no apparent reason why these supplements should be effective as ergogenic aids' (p. 304). The amounts given were far greater than those found in amino acid tablets and about the same as that in 100 grams of meat or chicken.

> Resistance-trained athletes may need more protein in their diet when attempting to increase lean muscle mass, but no reputable scientific evidence indicates that arginine, lysine, and ornithine supplementation provide any additional benefit.
>
> *M. H. Williams.*
> *The Ergogenics Edge (1998, p. 133)*

A study at the Australian Institute of Sport (Fricker, Beasley and Copeland 1988) showed that the best stimulation of growth hormone was exercising in the fasted state (no food for the previous eight hours). In this study throwers from the track and field team were divided into one of three trials. In one trial they took a commercial amino acid supplement with 1,800 milligrams of arginine and 1,200 milligrams of ornithine one hour before a weight training program, in another trial they had a normal breakfast and in a third trial they fasted. Those athletes who exercised in the fasted state showed the greatest increase in growth hormone levels. The addition of an amino acid supplement didn't enhance growth hormone release. Interestingly, even if a nutritional supplement does increase growth hormone, there is no evidence that the extra growth hormone increases muscle strength. As a result of this research, arginine, ornithine and lysine have gone out of favour with strength athletes in recent years, suggesting they had little to offer in the first place.

Bee Pollen

Bee pollen has been claimed to improve athletic and sexual performance, prevent infection and cancer, prolong life and improve digestion. Dr.

Melvin Williams said that 'six well-controlled studies reported that bee pollen supplementation had no effect on metabolic, physiological and psychological responses to exercise, $\dot{V}O_2$max, or endurance capacity in several exercise tasks' (1998, p. 135).

An advertisement for bee pollen states: 'Bee pollen contains more amino acids than any other natural substance and all the amino acids necessary for human beings. No other natural substance can make this claim'. Except, of course, milk, yogurt, cheese, meat, poultry, seafood and eggs.

> Bee pollen offers a glamorous and exotic approach to performance enhancement. However, there is doubt over the real composition of some supplements. This might explain why the controlled trials have failed to find any improvement after taking bee pollen. The balance of studies suggest there is no effect.
>
> *Dr. Louise Burke, Head of Sports Nutrition,*
> *Australian Institute of Sport (1995, p. 131)*

Because the digestibility of bee pollen is quite low, it is not a particularly useful food supplement. Athletes who are prone to allergies or with a known reaction to pollen are advised to avoid bee pollen. This supplement has been out of favour since the 1990s.

Carnitine

Carnitine came to prominence when Italy won the 1982 World Cup of soccer as their players were supposedly on carnitine. Was it the carnitine that led to success? It seems more likely that Italy won because they were the best team in the tournament.

Carnitine is made in the liver from the amino acids lysine and methionine and stored in the heart and muscles. Carnitine is also in red meat and some dairy foods, with the average non-vegetarian diet providing 100 to 300 milligrams of carnitine each day.

Carnitine is commonly marketed as useful for body fat loss and appears in most 'fat mobilisers' or 'fat metabolisers'. Carnitine is necessary for the transport of fat into the mitochondria, the powerhouses of body cells. The theory is that carnitine can mobilise more fat into the mitochondria so it can be used as fuel and improve endurance and increase the rate of body fat loss. Unfortunately, the theory is not supported by research. Just because you can fill the mitochondria with more fat doesn't mean that the mitochondria will burn more fat. Muscle appears to have enough natural carnitine to work at maximal rates anyway, and carnitine supplements don't increase muscle carnitine levels; the extra is merely excreted.

There is no evidence that the body's supply of carnitine becomes depleted in heavy exercise. Carnitine supplementation does not improve sports performance or help weight loss. Evidence does suggest that supplemental carnitine can improve the work capacity of people with stable angina, but that is hardly useful to fit athletes.

In their review of the scientific literature, Moffat and Chelland (in Wolinsky and Driskell 2004) concluded that 'the majority of studies reveal that carnitine supplementation does not seem to provide an ergogenic benefit to human performance' (p. 74).

And why is it called carnitine? Because no one can pronounce its real name: L-beta-hydroxy-gamma-N-trimethylaminobutyric acid.

Chromium and Chromium Picolinate

Chromium, a metal, is a part of the glucose tolerance factor that helps insulin to work effectively. As it also assists in protein metabolism, it got the attention of those wishing to increase muscle mass and strength. Sold mainly as chromium picolinate, it is also promoted as reducing body fat.

There is a patent for chromium picolinate. Being patented, however, doesn't mean that it is useful or meets its claims, just that it is different to other items. In 1997 the patent holders in the United States were ordered by the Federal Trade Commission to stop making weight loss claims as they could not be substantiated.

High-quality research studies found no indication of an ergogenic effect in athletes from chromium supplementation. A study of 36 American football players revealed that chromium picolinate supplements of 200 micrograms (mcg) a day had no effect on muscle mass or strength, nor reduced body fat levels (Clancy et al. 1994). This has been supported by all subsequent published research.

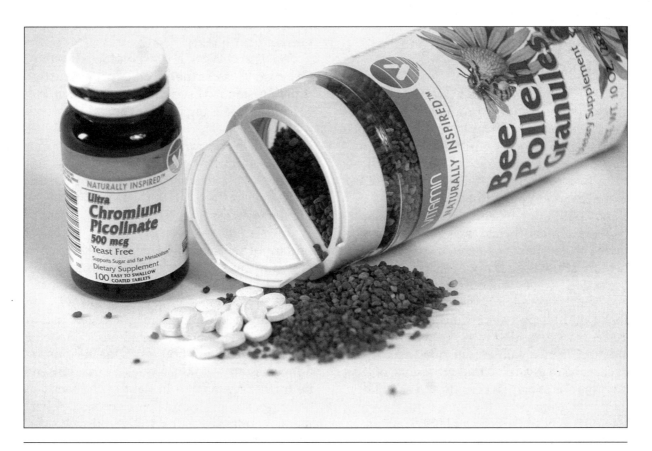

Supplements such as bee pollen and chromium picolinate are not recommended because they have no proven benefit for athletic performance.

The preponderance of evidence shows that chromium supplements will not increase lean body mass or decrease fat mass, despite the widespread hype to the contrary.

Dr. Priscilla Clarkson, University of Massachusetts, USA (1997, p. 347)

An adequate intake for chromium has been reliably estimated to be 35 micrograms for men and 25 micrograms for women. Good sources of chromium include meats, cheese, nuts, whole grains and brewers yeast. Chromium intakes of up to 400 micrograms daily don't appear to be toxic.

As with many essential minerals, chromium supplementation will be useful if the athlete has a diagnosed chromium deficiency. It appears that more chromium is lost in the urine during exercise than during rest days, but trained athletes may be able to conserve chromium better than nonathletes may. As yet, chromium deficiency has not been frequently measured in athletes. There is continuing research on chromium as an ergogenic aid, such as observing whether chromium helps shuttle glucose into active muscles during sprint work when given in a sports drink.

Coenzyme Q10, CoQ10 or Ubiquinone

CoQ10 is a molecule found in the mitochondria and is involved in ATP production, hence the theory that extra as a supplement will enhance sports performance. CoQ10 is also an antioxidant that soaks up the destructive free radicals in the body. Our bodies are able to make CoQ10, and even more comes in our food.

As CoQ10 supplements seemed to help heart patients improve their exercise tolerance, it was hoped that a similar effect would be seen with healthy athletes. This hope has not been substantiated by subsequent research on athletes. For healthy people, there is yet no evidence that CoQ10 supplements improves health or performance, or delays aging as some have claimed. In two studies, when triathletes and cyclists were given 100 milligrams of CoQ10 a day for four to eight weeks (Braun et al. 1991), or 1 milligram per kilogram of body weight for four weeks (Weston et al. 1997), it didn't improve their performance at all. The clinical application of CoQ10 is likely to be more useful than any sports nutrition application.

Fat Mobilisers, Fat Metabolisers and Fat Transporters

Fat mobilisers, fat metabolisers and fat transporters do not help body fat loss at all. The only way to mobilise fat is to exercise and eat fewer kilojoules than you burn. A tablet cannot get rid of body fat for you. Give them a miss; it's as simple as that. Most will contain carnitine, inositol, choline and other ingredients with no proven ability to assist fat loss.

Ginseng

The root of the plant *Panax ginseng* has been used in China as a tonic for centuries. Its active ingredients are steroid glycosides called ginsenosides. Obtaining authentic ginseng is difficult and expensive; hence, the amount of ginsenosides greatly varies in commercial preparations, some being found to have none at all.

Large doses of ginsenosides given to animals seem to increase endurance and promote muscle synthesis. This evidence has been hard to reproduce in human performance studies, possibly because commercial preparations of ginseng vary so much, and some research has been of poor quality.

Engels and Wirth (1997) conducted a study designed to assess the effects of providing two different standardised doses of *Panax ginseng* (200 mg and 400 mg per day) on graded maximal exercise. Thirty-six healthy men were involved in the randomised, double-blind, placebo-controlled trial for eight weeks. The habitual physical activity levels of the participants varied from the fairly sedentary to the regular exerciser.

Ginseng supplementation had no effect on any of the measured parameters: oxygen consumption, respiratory exchange ratio, blood lactate, heart rate and perceived exertion. Chronic ginseng consumption was not associated with a change in oxygen use or any improvement in aerobic work capacity. Despite a disappointing result for the ginseng advocates, the authors requested that ginseng be further researched in light of the fact that early researchers found some ergogenic effect using standardised doses. They also warned that larger doses of ginseng (around 3,000 mg of root material) can cause diarrhea, hypertension and insomnia.

In a comprehensive review, Bahrke and Morgan (2002) concluded that 'there is an absence of compelling research evidence regarding the efficacy of ginseng use for the purpose of improving physical performance in humans'. This, the authors believe, is because a lot of research has flawed methods and it is difficult to get supplement samples with a guaranteed level of ginseng. There may also be interactions between the diet and medications taken by athletes in the studies.

According to the U.S. Olympic Committee on Substance Abuse Research and Education, no scientific evidence supports the claim of performance enhancement for ginseng; hence, it is not banned by the International Olympic Committee.

Siberian ginseng is not ginseng at all; it is an entirely different plant called *Eleutherococcus senticosus*. There is no evidence that it is useful to athletes.

FINAL SCORE

- People vary greatly in their response to training, environmental conditions, psychological barriers and nutritional supplements, so it will always be difficult to assess the value of proposed ergogenic aids.

- Some products have proven ergogenic properties in some athletes under certain conditions. They are creatine, sports drinks, carbohydrate supplements, caffeine and bicarbonate.

- Based on current knowledge, the best regimen for achieving optimal performance is to avoid excess body fat, drink plenty of fluids to avoid dehydration and eat enough carbohydrate to fuel your training program. Most nutritional supplements will not enhance sports performance in well-nourished athletes.

- Be wary of the 'health assessment' or 'fitness program' that is designed to find faults in your health that can only be rectified by one or more supplements. Supplements are often better at making profits for their manufacturers than they are at enhancing sports performance.

- It is difficult to check the quantity and quality of the ingredients of many supplements that may contain 20 or more 'natural' ingredients. In many cases, no analytical methods exist for verifying the contents.

- Caveat emptor (let the buyer beware). The current climate is that manufacturers can make claims for products, leaving it up to scientists to spend years of research to determine whether they work, whether they are safe and what is the best dose if they do appear to work.

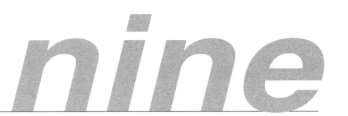

Food Choices for the Athlete's Kitchen

> It used to be standard practice that the pre-match meal consisted of eggs, steak and chicken. But I talked them into changing to complex carbohydrates. So now they will sup on porridge, pasta or wild rice.
>
> *Craig Johnston, Liverpool Football Club*

Craig Johnston was one of the athletes who adopted early the concept that good eating was a key to good performance. A crucial step to making wise food choices is understanding food labels. This chapter will arm you with the skills to decipher food labels (no easy task) and negotiate a supermarket. Even if you are already a skilled grocery shopper, you may get a few extra tips from this chapter.

Food Labels

Food labels are designed to get you to purchase the food. They will promote all the positive aspects, but may not mention some of the negative ones. Contrary to a popular viewpoint, food labels cannot lie to you, and very few do. They can, however, play on your emotions and word things to make you feel better about the product. For example, you

might see 'baked, not fried' on the label, suggesting that it is lower in fat. Often this means 'baked in a lot of fat, not fried in a lot of fat'. You see, the word *fried* is not good for sales. That's why, in the early 1990s, Kentucky Fried Chicken became KFC.

Many canned food labels state that they have no added preservatives, so you feel a warm glow when you purchase them. What they don't tell you is that canned foods do not require preservatives as canning is a means of preserving food in itself and has been for nearly 200 years. Although sugar and salt are preservatives, they may not come under the definition of a preservative in the food laws. For example, all canned food sold in Australia and New Zealand is preservative-free yet may still contain sugar and salt.

What Must Be on Food Labels?

Each label must include an ingredient list, the name and address of the manufacturer, distributor or importer, the weight or volume of the food, along with a description of what you can expect to find in the packet (see table 9.1). By law, the ingredients are listed on every food label in descending order—that is, the ingredient in the highest proportion is listed first. Some foods such as tea and coffee don't have to have an ingredient list. The only ingredient that doesn't have to be listed in descending order is water. The expression 'water added' may be placed at the end of the list.

Virtually all food labels now include a nutrition information panel (NIP) or a nutrition facts table. There are some exceptions: Bread bought fresh from a bakery, for example, can be sold without a wrapper. (The franchise bakers often will provide nutrition information on their range of products on request.)

By the way, if you want to convert kilojoules to kilocalories (we say calories for short), divide by four. If you want to be more accurate, divide by 4.18. There are quite a few pieces of information provided on a food label, and they are briefly described in table 9.1. When it comes to specific nutrient claims such as low fat or low salt, there are small differences between countries. These are detailed in table 9.2.

Nutrition Claims

Any label making a nutrition claim definitely has to provide a nutrition panel. The panel will include information on the protein, fat (including saturated fat), carbohydrate (including the sugar component), kilojoules or calories,

Table 9.1   What Is on Food Labels

On the food label	Explanation
Ingredients	Ingredients will be listed in descending order (most to least).
Manufacturer or distributor	Contact details of the manufacturer or distributor in the country of sale must be provided, should you wish to make an enquiry or complaint.
Nutrient panel	Virtually all labeled foods have a nutrition information panel (nutrition facts panel) providing the calories or kilojoules, protein, fat (including saturated fat), carbohydrate (including sugars) and sodium. In some countries, the amount of cholesterol and fibre is also provided.
	The panel should also give nutrient details for any nutrient claim; for example, if the food has been calcium fortified, the calcium content must be declared.
	Information is provided per serve and per 100 g (or 100 mL) in the UK, Australia and New Zealand, whereas just serve sizes are given in the United States and Canada.
Percentage of main characterising ingredient	In Australia and New Zealand the label should also state the percentage of the main characterising ingredients, such as the percentage of strawberry in strawberry yogurt. In the UK, strawberry yogurt can have a picture of strawberries on the label only if real strawberries are included in the ingredients; an artificially flavoured version cannot.
Percentage of daily values	In the United States, as well as the amount of each nutrient present, the percentage of the day's requirements for each nutrient is given based on a 2,000-calorie (8,400 kJ) or 2,500-calorie (10,450 kJ) diet. In the UK, guideline daily amounts are based on 2,000 calories for women and 2,500 calories for men. In both cases, they should not be confused with the recommended intakes of nutrients. In Canada, each vitamin or mineral listed will be shown as a percentage of the recommended daily needs.
Description of product	Well, you've got to know what you are buying (although it doesn't always look the same as the picture on the label).
'Use by' or 'best before' date	These dates can be on any food with a shelf life less than two years. Most foods will carry 'best before' dates. It doesn't mean that the food is 'off' once the date has passed by a day or two (usually it isn't if it has been stored correctly). The 'use by' date will be used mainly on foods that should not be consumed after that date for health reasons. Sometimes you may see a 'display until' date; this date is for shop staff and not the public. You should heed the 'use by' or 'best before' dates.

Table 9.2   Summary of Food Label Terms

On the food label	What does it mean?
Ingredients	The ingredients have to be listed in descending order (most to least) in all countries. The main characterising ingredients has to be given as a percentage in some countries, such as the percentage of apple in apple pie.
Made by	The address of the manufacturer, or the local distributor if the food was made in another country.
Reduced fat	The interpretation in most countries is that the amount of fat should be reduced by at least a quarter (25% reduction) compared to the standard food.
Low fat	Less than 3 g of fat per 100 g in solid foods and less than 1.5 g of fat in liquid food (Australia and New Zealand) Less than 3 g of fat per 100 g (UK) Less than 3 g of fat per serve (United States and Canada).
Fat free	Less than 0.15 g of fat per 100 g of food (Australia and New Zealand) Less than 0.15 g of fat per 100 g of food (UK) Less than 0.5 g of fat per serve (United States and Canada)
X% fat-free	Should be used only when a food is classified as low fat. For example, if a food is 97% fat-free, it will have no more than 3 g of fat in 100 g of food. X% fat-free claims cannot be made in the UK.
Low saturated fat	Less than 1.5 g saturated fat per 100 g of solid food and less than 0.75 g saturated fat per 100 g of liquid food. It must also comply with conditions for a low fat claim (Australia and New Zealand) Less than 1.5 g saturated fat per 100 g and not more than 10% of the kilojoules (calories) of the product (UK) Less than 0.5 g of saturated fat and less than 0.5 g trans fat per serve (United States and Canada)
Low cholesterol	Less than 20 mg cholesterol in 100 g (Australia, New Zealand and Canada) or in a serve (United States). In most countries you can make a low-cholesterol claim only on a food that is low in saturated fat. Check the label as there is little advantage in eating low-cholesterol foods that are high in saturated fat. There is no definition of low cholesterol in the UK and low cholesterol claims are no longer recommended.
Cholesterol-free	Less than 3 mg of cholesterol per 100 g and meet the conditions for low fat or saturated fat to be less than 20% of the total fat (Australia and New Zealand) Less than 3 mg of cholesterol and 2 g or less of saturated fat per serve (Canada) Less than 5 mg of cholesterol per 100 g (UK), although it is recommended that cholesterol-free claims no longer be made Less than 2 mg of cholesterol and 2 g or less of saturated fat per serve (United States)
Fibre	A high-fibre food will have: At least 3 g of fibre per serve (Australia and New Zealand) At least 4 g of fibre per serve (Canada) At least 4 g of fibre per 100 g (UK) At least 5 g of fibre per serve (United States)

(continued)

125

Table 9.2 *(continued)*

On the food label	What does it mean?
Low salt/sodium	Less than 120 mg of sodium per 100 g of food (Australia and New Zealand)
	Less than 40 mg of sodium per 100 g (UK and Canada)
	Less than 140 mg of sodium per 100 g (United States)
Salt reduced	The interpretation in most countries is that the amount of sodium has been reduced by at least a quarter (25% reduction)
Light, lite	This label should tell you what it is 'light' in, such as light in salt, light in colour. It may not be light in energy.
Low joule Calorie-free	Virtually free of kilojoules or calories
	Fewer than 80 kJ per 100 mL of liquid foods and fewer than 170 kJ per 100 g of solid or semisolid foods (Australia and New Zealand)
	Fewer than 1 cal per 100 g (Canada)
	Fewer than 40 cal per 100 g and fewer than 40 cal per serve (UK)
	Fewer than 5 cal per serve (United States)
No added sugar	No added sugars such as sucrose, glucose, dextrose, maltose, fructose, honey, molasses
Sugar-free	Less than 0.2 g of sugar per 100 g of solid food and less than 0.1 g of sugar per 100 g of liquid food (Australia and New Zealand)
	Only permitted on low-carbohydrate foods that have fewer than 1 cal per 100 g or 1 cal per 100 mL (Canada)
	Less than 0.2 g of sugar per 100 g (UK)
	Less than 0.5 g of sugar per serve (United States)
Natural	There is no definition for this term. Most manufacturers use the term to mean they have not used additives in the product.

sodium and other nutrients for which there has been a nutrient claim. For example, if the food label states that the food is a good source of fibre, then it must tell you how much fibre is present. Legal definitions do not exist for some of the nutrition claims on food labels, although this is under review in the United Kingdom, Australia and New Zealand.

Following are the nutrition claim recommendations of the Canadian Food Inspection Agency; the United States Food and Drug Administration; and the Ministry of Agriculture, Fisheries and Food (UK), as well as the recommendations in the Food Standards Australia New Zealand Code of Practice. Please note that they are only a summary—more comprehensive information can be accessed from government agencies in each country.

A reduced-fat or less-fat product must be at least 25 per cent lower in fat than the regular item. It doesn't mean it is 'low fat'. A food that would normally contain 40 grams of fat per 100 grams but is reduced to 30 grams of fat is 25 per cent lower in fat, but this is hardly low fat. If it were truly low in fat, it would be classified as a low-fat food, which is classified as follows:

- 3.0 grams of fat per 100 grams, or less, in a solid food and 1.5 grams of fat per 100 grams, or less, in a liquid food in Australia and New Zealand
- 3.0 grams of fat per 100 grams, or less, in the United Kingdom
- 3.0 grams of fat, or less, per serve in the United States and Canada

So, it follows that a 'reduced-fat' food may not be a 'low-fat' food.

You can see in table 9.2 that although fat-free foods can have some fat, the amounts that are allowed are next to nothing in fat terms. The same holds true for 'low saturated fat', which varies in different countries from 0.5 to 1.5

grams of saturated fat per serve or per 100 grams. Although each country has a different definition, the expression *low saturated fat* does indeed mean 'low in saturated fat'.

The expression 'X% fat-free' should be used only on foods that meet the requirements for 'low fat' or 'fat-free', and it must carry a statement of the total fat content (expressed as a percentage of the food) in close proximity to the claim. So, a food can be labeled as '97% fat-free', meaning it is 3 percent fat and therefore a low-fat food. This style of claim is no longer recommended for use in the United Kingdom.

A claim for low cholesterol can be made only if the cholesterol content is not more than 20 milligrams of cholesterol per 100 grams (in Australia, New Zealand and Canada) or not more than 20 milligrams per serve and not more than 2 grams of saturated fat per serve (in the United States). It can be a bit distracting because the cholesterol content of a food is not a major health issue; the type of fat has the biggest effect on health. It is for this reason that the Food Standards Agency in the United Kingdom recommends that low cholesterol claims no longer be made on food labels. The cholesterol content of a food is not related to its fat content. So, 'cholesterol-free' does not mean low in fat, and a cholesterol-free food can still be high in fat (e.g., cholesterol-free oils and potato crisps), so check the label. Any reference to cholesterol in Australia and New Zealand should be made only on a food that is either 'low fat' or not more than 20 per cent saturated fat.

In most Western countries, the term *cholesterol-free* means that the food will have an insignificant amount of cholesterol. The UK Food Standards Agency recommends that food labels no longer make any reference to cholesterol, while other countries stipulate that a cholesterol claim can only be made on a low saturated fat food. See table 9.2 for more specific details.

The fibre content can be a useful selling point. If the food is claimed to be 'high fibre', it will have around 3 to 5 grams of fibre per serve. Table 9.2 gives more details for each country. As adults should consume around 25 to 30 grams of fibre a day to avoid constipation and to keep the gut healthy, any food providing 4 grams of fibre in a normal serve size will help achieve your fibre needs. Some processed foods may add fibre to a product to meet the criteria for 'high fibre'.

There is a legal definition for a 'low-salt' food in most Western countries (table 9.2). Salt is sodium chloride, and it is the sodium component that is of most interest to us from a health perspective. Excessive sodium intake can raise blood pressure. When determining whether the food is low salt, you will need to check the label for the sodium level. Many food companies are now actively working to reduce the sodium levels of their products to give us more low-salt and salt-reduced choices.

A 'reduced-salt' food must be at least 25 per cent lower in sodium than the same quantity of the reference food. Salt is a learned taste and can often detract from the natural flavours of food (or mask the lack of flavour in food!). We generally consume far more salt than we need, so I suggest you choose lower salt foods.

The expression *light* or *lite* is not defined in any country, although the product should specify what it is referring to (e.g., light in flavour or texture). It does not necessarily mean the food is light in kilojoules or calories. For

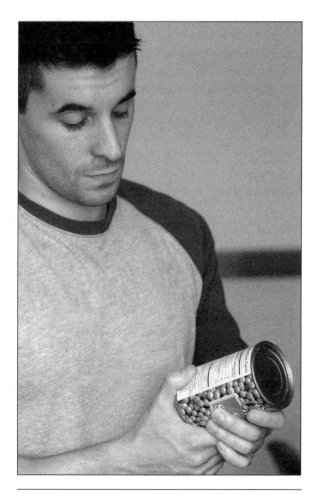

You can verify nutrition claims by carefully reading food labels.

example, light olive oil is only light in taste, and light potato crisps are reduced in salt, although often still high in saturated fat.

A low-kilojoule or calorie-free food is truly that—low in kilojoules or calories. Many low-kilojoule foods contain a sugar substitute such as aspartame (Nutrasweet). Eating low-kilojoule foods may make little difference to your weight or your appetite, so don't assume they will automatically result in weight loss. There is not a shred of evidence that any sugar substitute (artificial sweetener) causes cancer in the amounts consumed by humans. The rumour that Nutrasweet causes multiple sclerosis is one of the many e-mail nutrition hoaxes that make the rounds.

'No added sugar' means that the food manufacturer did not add sucrose, honey, glucose, molasses, malt, and so forth. Big deal. Sugar is not as evil as the pop nutritionists try to make it out to be. It doesn't give you pimples, heart disease, diabetes or in-growing toenails. Be mindful that 'no added sugar' foods may not be low in kilojoules, although they may have fewer kilojoules than the regular product with sugar. For example, a flavoured yogurt without sugar (artificially sweetened) will have fewer kilojoules than regular flavoured yogurt. Sugar is often replaced in confectionery (candy) and chewing gum by other sweetening agents to reduce the risk of tooth decay. Other than that, enjoy sugar if you wish and concentrate on

bigger nutrition issues, such as the type of fat, salt content, fibre levels and whether the food is a good source of other essential nutrients.

Natural is a great marketing word, but it has no legal definition under food law. Most companies use it to mean 'no additives' or 'minimally processed'. I suggest you read the ingredient list and see if it meets your definition of natural. (Note that beef fat and salt are 'natural'.)

Health Claims

At the time of writing only the United States and Canada permitted companies to print health claims on foods. For example, in Canada, foods with more than 5 per cent of the daily needs of iron can include the expression: 'This food is a good source of iron. Iron is a factor in red blood cell formation'. The idea of health claims on food labels is under consideration in the United Kingdom, Australia and New Zealand. A health claim establishes a relationship between a nutrient or food ingredient and a specific disease or health condition. This relationship must have been clearly identified through scientific studies. For example, a food label might state that 'This food is high in calcium. A diet rich in calcium is linked to a reduced risk of osteoporosis'. The food cannot imply, however, that it is an essential food, nor that it has the ability to forestall osteoporosis,

Web Sites About Food Labeling

For more information on food labeling, see the following sites:

Australia and New Zealand

www.foodstandards.gov.au/whatsinfood/foodlabelling.cfm

United Kingdom

www.food.gov.uk/foodlabelling/

www.nutrition.org.uk

United States

www.cfsan.fda.gov/~dms/foodlab.html

Canada

www.inspection.gc.ca/english/toc/labetie.shtml

as it is the overall diet that influences disease, not specific foods.

Shopping Tips

Some simple tips can make you a more efficient and wiser grocery shopper. Naturally, you may already have shopping down to an art form, but those who still have some difficulty may find the tips useful.

Low Fat

As a general guide, a food needs to be less than 10 per cent fat before it can be considered relatively low in fat. In other words, it must have less than 10 grams of fat per 100 grams of food. (In reality, a food must be less than 3 per cent fat to be called low fat, but nutritionally, foods consisting of less than 10 per cent fat are considered low in fat.) Many foods are fat-free, such as fruit, vegetables, pasta and rice. Bread and breakfast cereals generally have little fat. But don't use it as law because some nutritious foods are more than 10 per cent fat, such as avocado, nuts, peanut butter and good-quality chocolate.

What Type of Fat?

Saturated, monounsaturated and polyunsaturated are all types of fat. The unsaturated versions are generally the healthier choices as they don't raise blood cholesterol, but remember that all fat is high in energy, so you will need to use it wisely. Be aware that any reference to the cholesterol content (e.g., cholesterol-free) may not be linked to the amount of fat in that product. For example, vegetable oils will be cholesterol-free, yet will also be 100 per cent fat and high in kilojoules.

Salt of the Earth

Most people will benefit from eating less salt than they currently do. About 75 per cent of our salt intake comes from foods in which the manufacturer has added salt, so not adding salt to your dinner doesn't mean you are on a low-salt diet. I recommend you choose the salt-reduced or low-salt versions of food so that you taste the taste rather than the salt. A high salt intake is linked to high blood pressure and excess calcium loss from the bones.

Go Fruity

Buy and eat plenty of fresh fruit. Fruit is a great source of carbohydrate, fibre, water and antioxidants. Canned fruits are also nutritious and are great for dessert or on breakfast cereal.

Frozen Assets

Frozen foods are exceptionally convenient, especially for single people or couples. Frozen vegetables are very nutritious with only minor nutrition loss during the blanching before freezing. (Blanching is the process of dipping into boiling water for a short time.) Don't for a moment think that frozen vegetables are less nutritious than fresh. In fact, they may be more nutritious if you have left your fresh vegetables too long before you get around to eating them. Also, check your frozen meals for their nutrition profile. Many will promote their benefits, such as being low in fat, but you will need to check that they are also a reasonable source of fibre (6+ grams of fibre for a medium meal would be expected) and are not too high in sodium (I suggest less than 300 milligrams for a medium meal).

Very, Very Rice

Asian meals are usually good value for health. Stock up on rice and vegies for a stir-fry high in carbohydrate. Add some lean meat, chicken or seafood for protein, iron and zinc.

Pasta Blasta

Pasta can be the base of so many simple and inexpensive meals. The carbohydrate is great for replacing glycogen stores. There are lots of pasta sauces on the market—just add your own extra vegetables for fibre and antioxidants.

Simple Fare

Buy a precooked chicken, take it home, remove the skin and serve with microwaved vegetables. Or get a low-fat frozen meal from the supermarket; add extra potato, vegetables or rice if it doesn't look filling enough. Or buy a prepackaged rice or pasta dish. Check the label to make sure you aren't getting too much fat or salt. Simplicity is the friend of the tired and hungry athlete.

Lunch Cereals

Who said that breakfast cereals should be eaten only at breakfast? Cereal and milk are great any time of the day, and are popular with young athletes after school, providing valuable carbohydrate, protein, fibre, vitamins and minerals.

Oooh Yeah!

If your baseline diet is good, there will always be room for some of your very favourite foods such as ice cream, chocolate, confectionery and pizza. Two things to keep in mind regarding these foods are balance and moderation.

FINAL SCORE

- Familiarity with your local supermarket will make shopping easy and quick.
- A simple knowledge of food labels allows you to compare products and helps you make more nutritious choices.
- If you forget everything else, always remember to choose the week's groceries with the view to keeping the saturated fat and salt to a minimum.
- The least processed foods are generally the most nutritious.

Meal Tips for Restaurants and Road Trips

ten

> When we went on the road, we ate as a team, so I had to eat the Japanese stuff. All kinds of stuff: moving stuff, live stuff, stinky stuff, ugly stuff. I talked to the interpreter to make sure they had some fried chicken or else I would have starved.
>
> *Brian Williams, Chicago Cubs baseball pitcher on his return from a season in Japan (2000)*

It is not always convenient to prepare all your own meals and snacks. Often you will have to eat on the road, at airport terminals or at restaurants. Sometimes, like Brian Williams quoted above, you may have to make arrangements to have your style of food available. It is still important that you keep to your nutrition goals for optimal performance. This chapter is a guide to making the best choices when you cannot prepare your own meals.

Snacks

Your mother was right—one of the best snack foods is a piece of fruit for its carbohydrate, fibre and antioxidants, all at a very good price. The only thing going against fruit is that it doesn't always travel well on hot days and can be easily bruised. This can be overcome by storing it in a cooler bag. Another snack favourite with athletes is the food bar, and a great variety is available. Many of them are low in total fat and saturated fat. If nuts or seeds are added, the fat content will rise. Of course, these are healthy ingredients, and their fat is mainly unsaturated.

Some snacks will have added sugar to improve the taste, thus raising the carbohydrate content. This should not cause alarm as fit people can afford some kilojoules as sugar, and the extra carbohydrate will be burned during training and sport.

Table 10.1 provides a brief guide to the most common snacks.

Take-Aways

With some smart thinking you can choose a better class of take-away, which includes fast food and carry-out food. Some are not the perfect choice, but in a tight situation they can still keep you on track for a good dose of your daily carbohydrate and essential nutrient needs. Many franchised take-aways are now offering salad bars, fruit, vegetarian meals and a range of low-fat choices. Importantly, most of the franchised chains provide the nutrition profiles online or in-store for their entire menu. Check the profiles to identify the lower fat and lower salt choices. Check the energy (kJ or cal) content if you are watching your waistline.

Table 10.1 Snack Guide

Food	Higher nutritional value	Lower nutritional value
Fruit	The fastest food around. Choose your favourite. Canned fruit and dried fruit are also good choices.	Fruit juice because of minimal fibre (however, still a good source of carbohydrate and water).
Food bars	There are low-fat versions of fruit bars, muesli bars, sports bars and breakfast bars. Recommend less than 4 g fat and more than 20 g carbohydrate per food bar weighing 30–45 g.	Coated food bars such as yogurt and chocolate coating as they usually have a high saturated fat coating (i.e., are often not real yogurt or real chocolate).
Milk	Flavoured milk. (Most flavoured milks are based on reduced-fat milk. Sure, they have some sugar, but not enough to diminish the value of the milk nutrients.) Reduced-fat and nonfat milk. Add some fruit or flavouring for carbohydrate and taste.	Full-cream milk (still nutritious, but higher in fat).
Bread and bread rolls	Fruit bread rolls with dried fruit. Whole-grain breads as they have fibre—they take longer to chew and are more filling. Bread rolls, Lebanese bread, pita bread, Turkish bread.	Rolls with cheese, bacon and other savoury flavourings. White breads. Croissants.
Muffins	Plain English muffins to which you can add your own spread. Sweet muffins.	Savoury muffins with fatty ingredients.
Nuts	Plain, unsalted.	Roasted and salted.
Take-aways	See Dining Out Guide (table 10.2) later in chapter.	
Sandwiches	See Dining Out Guide (table 10.2) later in chapter.	

Still Number 1

The most popular take-away of all time is the sandwich or bread roll. Ask for little or no margarine and get them to reduce the fatty fillings such as cheese. Lean fillings with plenty of salads is the best way to go.

Fowled Out

Take a precooked chicken home, remove the skin and serve with microwaved starchy vegetables or salad and bread. The breast meat is lowest in fat. A dead-easy meal.

Rice Is Nice

Steamed rice is available from every Asian or Chinese take-away. Make sure this carbohydrate source dominates the plate, then add some lean meat or seafood for protein, and some vegetables. You can add a steamed spring roll for variety.

Veg Out

Any meal that is high in vegetables is likely to have less fat and more carbohydrate. Corn and peas are filling, low in fat and high in carbohydrate. Don't add butter or margarine if you need to restrict your fat intake. Ask for plenty of vegetables, or vegetable-based foods, when getting a take-away (but not just hot chips and fries!).

Pasta Lasta Longa

Pasta is always a favourite with athletes. Make sure you get a big serve, and ask them to reduce the oil. The topping is crucial—a tomato- or seafood-based sauce will have less fat. Remember, only a sprinkle of cheese on top.

Pie-Eyed

Meat pies and pork pies are still popular in Australia and the United Kingdom, but they are changing. Lower-fat types are becoming available, and although lower in fat than in the past, they aren't a great source of carbohydrate. Athletes will need to supplement with fruit, fruit juice or a fruit bun. Some vegetarian pasties are a good choice.

Chewing Your Spud

The baked potato is back! Try toppings such as baked beans, coleslaw and creamed corn. Go light on the cheese topping. A great, inexpensive meal.

Pizza Hit

The best pizza choices are the thick-crust type with a vegetarian or seafood topping. You could ask for less cheese to get the fat content even lower. Beware of fatty toppings such as cabanossi and other fatty meats.

Remove the Fat of the Land

Try removing the following from take-away foods:

- Skin from chicken
- Batter from fish
- Excess fat from meat

Tijuana Tucker

If you go Mexican, aim for a burrito or enchilada with salad, lean meat, chicken or beans. Corn chips with cheese and sour cream may

taste great, but they have a lot more fat than carbohydrate.

Lebanese, Please

You might have to do some negotiating here. Kebabs, cabbage rolls, tabouleh, vegetarian kibbi and flat bread are the best choices. Beware of any dish that's fried or deep-fried. Often you can choose 'wet' dishes made from potatoes, beans, lentils or rice. Hummus and baba ghannouj are popular. Eat these with plenty of rice or bread.

Salad Days

The popularity of the salad bar is on the rise. The response to the obesity issue has meant that many take-away outlets now offer fresh fruit and a range of salads. Some offer you a decent breakfast too. Take advantage of this trend.

Have the Day Off!

There is no harm in eating the occasional fatty meal, especially if you are more than a couple of days away from competition. Make sure your eating habits improve before the big event. The more often you stray from wholesome eating, the more likely you will be to deep-fry your chances of success. It's your decision.

Tips for Dining Out

More and more restaurants now offer lower-fat, 'light' meals to patrons, making it a little easier to eat well away from home. Here are some simple tips to make dining out fit into your health and performance goals. Enjoy the experience. The information is summarised in table 10.2.

Waitresses Don't Bite!

Feel comfortable asking the waiting staff for information about the menu. Ask them to make simple changes if possible: 'The grilled fish is fine, but please leave off the butter sauce'. Beware of the 'grease factor'. Cheese, cream and oil can add lots of fat to a meal.

Be Fruitful

Eat one or two pieces of fruit before you go out. Then you won't arrive at the restaurant so hungry that you forget all your good intentions.

Get Wet

Ask for a jug of water to quench your thirst before you order other drinks. Drink water, mineral water, juice or a soft drink between alcoholic drinks. Drink alcohol sparingly— remember that it's a dehydrating fluid.

Read That Menu

Descriptions that include the words *pan-fried, butter sauce, cream sauce, sautéed, fried, battered* and *creamed* are dead giveaways for a high-fat meal. It's easy to ask for the sauce to be left off.

Beware the Smorgasbord Monster!

A smorgasbord demands that you have a little bit of everything until your plate is so loaded you can't see the first three selections you made. This can easily lead to overeating. So, try three or four choices at first and go back for more later if you're still hungry. The key is self-control and self-respect.

Well Bread

Many athletes will eat more food than sedentary people will. The bread roll is a useful adjunct to any athlete's meal. Ask for extra bread rolls if necessary, especially if the meal has been delayed and will be served well past

your usual eating time. Bread can also supplement a low-carbohydrate meal.

Salacious Salads and Voracious Vegetables

Salad bars are usually inexpensive. Very active people can fill up on salads made from rice, pasta, potato or beans for a carbohydrate base. Order salads without oil and fatty dressings. Although side salads are very nutritious, they are generally low in carbohydrate. If the main course comes with vegetables, ask for extra potato, peas and corn to meet your carbohydrate needs.

Welcome Asia

Asian meals are always a good value for health. Get plenty of steamed rice, stir-fried vegetables, lean meat or seafood. Ask for extra steamed rice if you are hungry, but don't fill up on greasy food.

What's Your Perspective?

If you have been eating plenty of carbohydrate at breakfast and lunch, then don't be fanatical about the carbohydrate in an occasional meal out. For example, a meal of grilled fish and salad is good nutrition and although it is low in carbohydrate, you may have made up for this earlier in the day. Life and sport are meant to be enjoyed. Just make sure that you eat plenty of carbohydrate at the next meal and in the two days before sports events.

Table 10.2 Dining Out Guide

Food	Higher nutritional value	Lower nutritional value
Sandwiches and rolls	Fillings: Lean meat, salmon, tuna, chicken breast, turkey, baked beans, banana, cottage cheese, ricotta, salad vegetables. Go easy on the margarine or butter. Whole-meal roll if possible.	Fillings: luncheon meats (e.g., salami), hard cheese, cream cheese, sausages.
Chicken	Remove skin and stuffing. Breast meat is lowest in fat.	Deep fried, battered or crumbed pieces. Chicken nuggets.
Burgers	Hamburgers with grilled meat patty and lots of salad.	Burgers with fried meat patties, cheese and bacon. Battered and deep-fried fillings.

Food	Higher nutritional value	Lower nutritional value
Chips, fries	Smallest serve with the biggest chips/fries! (Big chips/fries have a lower fat content.)	Thin chips, fries, wedges. Thin chips have more fat.
Pizza	Vegetarian, lean meat or seafood topping; minimal cheese.	Fatty toppings such as salami, bacon, cabanossi, cheese. Garlic bread.
Pastries, pies	Pasties, pies and shepherd's pies, and other pastries with less than 10% fat (10 g per 100 g).	Pies, pasties, croissants, sausage rolls, hot dogs, chips, any deep-fried foods.
Seafood	Grilled fish, steamed shellfish and seafood.	Battered fish. Cream and fatty sauces.
Indian and Asian	Steamed rice, vegetable-based dishes, lean meat, seafood, clear soups, noodles, steamed spring rolls and steamed dim sims, dhal, lentils, curries (minimal fat), naan bread.	Fried rice or fried noodles, deep-fried and battered dishes such as sweet and sour pork, duck. Fried dim sims, excess satay sauce.
Lebanese	Souvlakia, kebabs, flat bread, salad, cabbage roll, tabouleh, vegetarian kibbi, lady fingers.	Felafel, fried kibbi, hummus and baba ghannouj (all nutritious but moderate fat). Any fried or high-oil food.
Italian	Pasta with tomato, seafood or pesto sauce—low oil, minestrone soup, plain bread, salad, pizza with minimal fat such as vegetarian or seafood.	Lasagne; cannelloni; cream, butter and cheese sauces such as alfredo; garlic bread; pizza with fatty meats and excess cheese.
Mexican	Taco, burrito or enchilada with salad; fish, lean meat, chicken, beans; gazpacho; salsa.	Dishes with cheese, sour cream or refried beans; nachos; corn chips.
Salad bars	All salads, vinaigrette dressing, fruit salad, whole-meal bread, baked potato, corn cobs.	High-fat salad dressings and mayonnaise, cream, sour cream.
Potato	Baked potato (minimum sour cream or cheese). Toppings: baked beans, cottage cheese, coleslaw, avocado and tomato, creamed corn.	Hot chips, french fries (wedges are a better choice). Potato cakes, potato scallops.
Family restaurant	See advice for above foods. Most soups are also low in fat. Fruit salad and fruit platter for dessert.	See advice for above foods.
Drinks	Water, mineral water and diet soft drinks are the best choices if you are controlling body fat.	Regular soft drinks, fruit juice, sensible amounts of alcohol.
Dessert	Low-fat frozen yogurt, fruit salad, low-fat ice cream.	Sweet pastries, cakes, ice cream.

On-the-Road Nutrition

Eating while on the road is a very personal affair, as demonstrated in the opening quote of the chapter. Travelling to compete in sport usually signals the culmination of all your training.

Unfortunately, travel can often mean delays, different time zones, take-away or restaurant foods and uncomfortable beds. Whether you're travelling overseas or interstate, or spending a couple of hours in the car, your aim is to arrive as fresh as a gazelle, ready to produce the performance of a lifetime. Following are some tips to maintain your nutrition goals when travelling. You may already be happy with what you arrange to eat. The following may help you to refine your food choices to get the best out of your body while on your travels.

Plan Ahead

If possible, travel so that you can keep close to your normal routine and try to avoid travel that causes you to rise too early or stay up too late. This becomes more important when you're flying.

Take Your Own Feed Bag

You might decide to bring your own meals rather than rely on hotels and take-aways. Grab your own breakfast cereal and milk (there are reduced-fat versions of powdered milk and UHT milk—ideal if you don't have refrigeration). Breakfast bars, muesli bars, fruit bars, Sustagen Sport, fresh fruit, dried fruit, canned fruit and fruit juice all travel well.

Minimise the Strain

Long hours of travel can upset your digestive system. Low-fibre meals, combined with being seated for long hours, can block your down-pipe. To minimise constipation, eat fibre-rich foods such as fresh fruit, fruit salad, wholemeal bread, breakfast cereals and vegetables.

Don't Starve

When travelling by car, bus or train, don't let yourself get too hungry or the first fast-food outlet you see might tempt you to make less-than-wise choices. Take some snacks with you such as fruit, sandwiches and low-fat muesli bars.

Don't Overeat

Because you are not active when you travel, you need less food than on training days. Don't confuse boredom with hunger or you will overeat—a big problem in sports with a weight limit. Some major event venues pro-

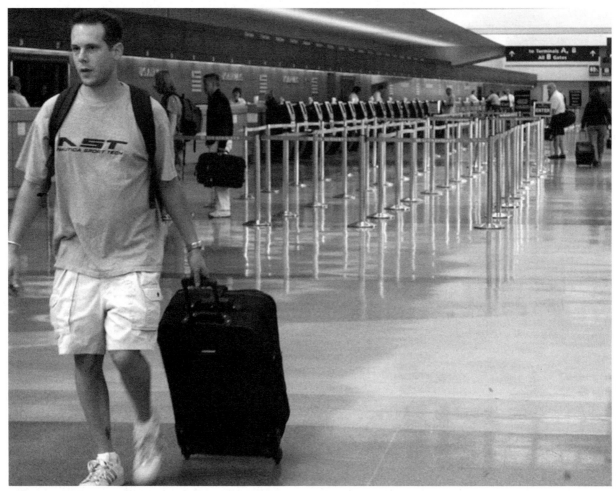

When travelling, do all you can to keep your food choices healthy and similar to what you would eat at home.

vide athletes with unlimited amounts of a big range of food, which makes it very easy to eat more than normal. You will need to consciously control your eating.

Feast Without Fear

You may have to eat lots of meals from restaurants and take-aways when on the road. Ask for plenty of steamed rice, pasta, bread or potatoes to provide enough carbohydrate, with vegetables and fruit for fibre. See table 10.2 for more ideas on the best choices when on the road.

This Is No Holiday

Travelling for competition can often take on a holiday atmosphere, pushing good nutrition to one side. Your goal is still to eat mainly wholesome, unprocessed foods. Ask the people serving you for assistance when choosing from a menu. It's no problem for them to go light on the margarine or hold the cheese sauce.

Avoiding Jet Lag

Airline travel can be arduous. On long trips that cross time zones, your 24-hour biological time clock, or circadian rhythm (from *circa diem*, Latin for 'about 24 hours'), becomes disrupted. This condition is called circadian dysrhythmia, or jet lag.

More than 300 bodily functions occur in a 24-hour rhythm. These functions normally have 'high' and 'low' points during the 24-hour period, corresponding to a sleep–wake cycle. For example, body temperature (which peaks at around 6 p.m.), heart rate (which is higher in the afternoon) and the stomach (which empties more quickly in the morning than in the evening) all have a circadian rhythm. Your performance can be affected by this sleep–wake cycle. Most people seem to be at their peak between 11 a.m. and 4 p.m., so it is no surprise that most world records are set in the afternoon.

Your circadian rhythm resynchronises at a rate of around 90 minutes a day after westward travel across time zones, and 60 minutes a day after eastward travel. This helps explain why jet lag seems more apparent after travelling east, when we 'lose time' and the body clock resynchronises more slowly, than it is after travelling west, when we 'gain time'.

Change Your Body Clock Time

When travelling across time zones, some people adjust their body clocks to their destination time in the two or three days before departure. On arrival they can quickly adopt local times for eating and sleeping. If you travel across time zones for only a day or two, keep to your regular home time zone so you don't try to change your body clock twice in 48 hours.

When travelling to another country, the first thing to do on arrival is to forget what time it is in your home country. As soon as you get on the plane, set your watch for the time in the country of destination and start thinking like a local. Experiment and find out what is comfortable to you.

Be an Early Bird

If possible, arrive at your destination well before the event to allow time for your body to adjust to the new time. As a guide, arrive one day early for every time zone crossed; that is, arrive three days early to adjust for a three-hour time difference. For international travel crossing six or more time zones, athletes seem to return to their peak within four to seven days, so allow a week in your new country before competition. Of course, not everyone has this luxury.

Acclimatise

If you are travelling from a cool climate to a warm one, it can take 7 to 10 days for your body to acclimatise to the warmer weather. Your sweat and general cooling physiology take a little time to get used to the higher temperature. Sweat will have a higher sodium level initially; then the sodium levels drop to adjust to the warmer weather and the need to conserve sodium. To speed up the acclimatisation, exercise in warmer conditions before you leave home. Some athletes do this inside with the heater on or by wearing extra clothing during training.

Go Low Fat

Contact the airline two days before departure to see whether they can cater for special meals. Most airlines will provide low-fat meals, your best choice, or vegetarian meals. Some airlines are so accustomed to working with sports teams and athletes that they even offer a high-carbohydrate athletes' meal. The bonus is that you tend to get served first! Some airlines are happy to provide extra bread and fruit for the hungry athlete. Teams can negotiate special arrangements with airlines.

Soak It Up

Keep up the nonalcoholic fluids. The humidity in an aircraft is around 10 to 15 per cent, which means that moisture is literally drained from your body. Drink mineral water, soft drinks or fruit juices when travelling by air. Bringing your own water bottle on long flights is a great idea. Tea and coffee can also be a part of your fluid intake as four to five cups in a flight hydrates the body equally as effectively as water. Give alcohol a miss as it dehydrates the body.

Stretch It Out

While flying, occasionally get up and do some stretches, especially during flights that are longer than two hours. This also helps keep you alert and relieves the monotony. Airlines now advise stretching and wriggling your toes and feet to minimise the risk of deep vein thrombosis (DVT). You can also try walking up and down the aisles to improve the blood flow in your legs. Try a quick wash near the end of the flight to freshen up.

Loosen Up

Your feet tend to swell on long flights, so wear comfortable shoes that can be easily loosened or removed, such as runners. Wear loose clothing and avoid anything that will dig into your body.

Zoom With a View

I prefer a window seat. That way, no one has to climb over me if I'm having a snooze. Others prefer an aisle seat as they can stretch their legs and get up whenever they please. Nobody fancies the middle seat! In some aircraft there is more leg room near the exit doors. If you are a frequent flyer, then seating arrangements can be made to suit you.

Make It a Good Night

Being on the road can play havoc with your sleeping habits. Changes in time zones, a different bed and pillow, unusual noises outside and different weather conditions all play their part in disrupting your sleep. To improve your chances of getting a good night's sleep, try these tips:

- Go for a light training session, or a good walk, about three hours before bedtime.
- Eat a high-carbohydrate snack before bedtime. It increases brain serotonin, which may help you to sleep.
- Keep the bedroom cool. Warm rooms can upset the sleep cycle.
- Don't nap during the day; you may not get to bed tired enough to sleep.
- Regulate your sleeping habits to local time as soon as possible.

Food Safety

When at home, you probably wash your hands before you prepare food, make sure all perishable foods are stored in the refrigerator and don't use foods past their 'use by' dates. When you are away from home, you often have to trust that your meals have been made under hygienic conditions. Your trust will be well placed in virtually all quality airlines, hotels and restaurants. In some countries and in some food outlets, however, it is wise to take precautionary measures to avoid food poisoning.

Avoiding Food Poisoning

When travelling for competition, you don't want to be laid low with a bout of food poisoning. Here are some simple guidelines on food and drink safety:

- If you are not sure of the quality of the local water supply, use bottled, boiled or sterilised water for drinks and teeth brushing. Avoid ice, mixed drinks, and foods washed in local water.
- If you are not sure of food preparation cleanliness, avoid raw foods, including unpeeled fruits and vegetables, washed salads, shellfish and so forth.
- Avoid undercooked meat or unpasteurised milk products.
- Avoid buying foods from local stalls and markets, where hygiene may be poor.
- Look for food that is well cooked and served hot (not warm).
- Avoid food from buffets that is not served very hot or chilled, or you suspect has been there for a long time.
- Consider taking live cultures (acidophilus, bifidus) or cultured yogurt with you as a preventative measure. Eat these if you do get food poisoning as they will help your bowels restock with healthier bacteria.

FINAL SCORE

- Be prepared to ask questions about the choices at take-aways and restaurants. With more knowledge, you can make wiser decisions.
- Download nutrient profiles of menu items from franchise restaurants' Web sites so you can identify the best choices.
- Generally, the lower fat, higher carbohydrate, least processed choices are the most nutritious and best suited to an athlete's needs.
- Plan ahead for travel. The quicker you can adapt to local conditions, the quicker you will recover from the lethargy of travelling.
- Consider food safety when travelling to other countries to reduce any chance of food poisoning.

part III

Weight Management for Athletes

eleven

Muscle Building and Weight Gain Strategies

> So I started my final diet. On Sunday and Monday I ate the new diet, labored strenuously through my workouts, and slept like a baby. But by Tuesday, without adequate fuel, I began to lag. My two egg whites for breakfast were hardly enough. I worked out in the morning listlessly. . . . I was so weak that even when I halved the amount of weight I normally pushed, I barely got through the workout.
>
> *Sam Fussell, bodybuilder, in* Muscle

Every elite athlete, and many recreational athletes, now weight train to increase muscle strength and muscle mass. Formerly the domain of male athletes, strength training is becoming a useful part of women's sport training. Good nutrition can help, but we have to look beyond the hype and find what is scientifically proven to help the strength athlete and those looking for greater muscle mass. Certainly, the Spartan diet followed by bodybuilder Sam Fussell may have been high in protein, but it lacked the carbohydrate to fuel his workouts. There is a smarter and healthier way to eat when trying to bulk up.

Formula for Strength and Muscle Bulk

To have the best chance to gain extra muscle, you need to have the basics in place first: the right genes, weight training, good nutrition and patience. These are discussed in the following sections.

The Right Genes

All athletes can increase their strength, but not all will find it easy to naturally increase muscle bulk. Take a look at your blood relatives, especially those of the same gender as you. If they were skinny at a similar age, then you may find it a little tougher to gain muscle mass. If your immediate relatives are solidly built, you will have a better chance of being able to pack on more muscle. The good news is that, independent of your genetics, you can always increase muscular strength with weight training even if the increase in muscle size is not spectacular.

Women will have more difficulty gaining muscle mass because of their lower levels of the hormone testosterone. A woman will notice a change in shape, definition, firmness and strength more than a change in muscle mass. Men have more testosterone and larger muscle fibres, a combination that gives them bigger muscles than women. Most women, with the exception of female bodybuilders, will prefer muscle strength over bulk. They can achieve this by following the nutrition guidelines in this chapter and engaging a strength and conditioning coach.

Weight Training

Muscles get bigger and stronger only if you use them. Nothing else will make them bigger. Amino acids won't make them bigger. Protein powders won't make them bigger. More muscle mass requires resistance exercise such as swimming (for the upper body), cycling (for the legs) or weight training. Get some professional advice on the best resistance exercise for you.

Good Nutrition

If you want to gain muscle, you have to eat good-quality food. You will need adequate protein and carbohydrate. The right amount of protein is quite easy to get. The average athlete already eats more protein than needed for weight training. (Your protein needs are covered in chapter 2.) Your meals have to have a reasonable amount of carbohydrate to fuel the muscles so they can do a longer and more efficient workout to increase muscle mass. Otherwise, you will feel like Sam Fussell quoted at the beginning of the chapter.

When you put muscle under stress through weight training, long-distance running or sprint sessions, a small amount of muscle damage occurs naturally. This is not cause for alarm because with time and healthy eating, the body will repair the damage. If you can eat enough protein and carbohydrate to minimise muscle breakdown, then it makes sense that you can gain muscle mass more quickly through training. Some supplements are thought to help reduce muscle damage, thereby enhancing muscle gain. Beware of faulty claims of supplements. You can read more about supplements later in this chapter and in chapter 8.

Patience

Creating bigger muscles takes time and effort. Although it happens more quickly in some than in others, it's likely to take 6 to 12 months to achieve significant gains in muscle size, even if you work hard at it. Realistic gains will be

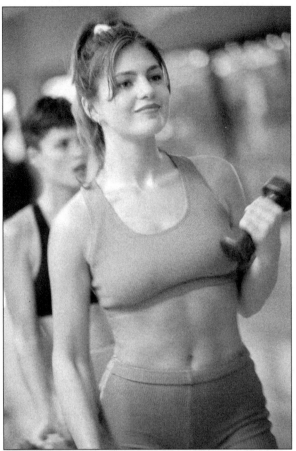

© Eyewire

To add muscle, you'll need to do resistance training and eat proper amounts of carbohydrate and protein.

between 0.2 and 1.0 kilogram (0.4 and 2.2 lb) per week. The rate of weight gain is usually faster in the first months and slows down thereafter. Hence, an athlete might gain 3 kilograms (6.6 lb) in the first month of weight training, but gain only 1 kilogram (2.2 lb) in the fourth month.

The remainder of the chapter focuses on nutrition and bulking up. I'll leave it to you to organise your own weight training program and to address the issue of patience. There's nothing you can do about your genes.

Who Can Benefit From Gains in Muscle and Weight?

Generally, four kinds of people want to increase their muscle mass for specific health or sports benefits.

• **Skinny people.** Some people are naturally lean and feel it is a disadvantage in sport and life. Gains in muscle mass may be slow, but gains in muscle strength can be significant. With a little extra muscle mass they are likely to get more respect in sport and on the street.

• **Unintentional weight losers.** Some athletes find it hard to maintain their weight as a sporting season progresses. This is common in football and rowing, in which training demands are heavy and the kilojoules going in don't match those going out. They need to eat more kilojoules to maintain their weight.

• **Set position athletes.** Some positions in team sports require strength and bulk, whereas others might rely on speed and additional muscle bulk slows them down. Those athletes who need extra muscle mass will need to adjust their diet and put in some extra time at the gym.

• **Unfit and overweight people.** Increasingly, unfit people are turning to weight training as a means to lose body fat and increase bone density. Older people now attend gyms because they know that weight training slows down osteoporosis and makes them less prone to falls and heart disease. Rather than building muscle mass, their primary goals are muscle growth, bone density and fat burning.

Although people often ask me how they can gain weight, what they really want to know is how they can increase muscle mass without increasing body fat. This can be difficult, especially if genetics has designed someone to be very lean. The nutrition tips provided in the next section can help increase muscle mass through weight training.

Nutrition for Bulking Up and Gaining Weight

Following the nutrition guidelines outlined in this section, in conjunction with a weight training program, will enable you to get maximal gains in muscle size. A summary of these guidelines is given in table 11.1. Based on all the scientific research, it is very unlikely that you will need more than 2 grams per kilogram of body weight of protein daily. If your training sessions are strenuous, you may need more than 8 grams of carbohydrate per kilogram of body weight. The fat guideline given in table 11.1 is more for general good health than for any training benefits. If you eat more fat than suggested, make sure it is mainly unsaturated fat. Nutritional supplements *may* help you, but you should read chapter 8 carefully before you spend any money on them.

Eat Adequate Protein

There is no doubt that athletes need greater amounts of protein than sedentary people do. Certainly, strength athletes and those doing resistance exercise need extra protein. However, it doesn't follow that they need a protein supplement. A high-quality diet with plenty of carbohydrate will almost always meet the protein needs of an athlete. (The protein needs of athletes is discussed in chapter 2.)

Athletes doing weight training will often find that protein supplements help increase muscle mass. Usually, they could have taken extra carbohydrate and achieved the same result. Why? Because the extra protein in the

Table 11.1 Nutrition for Increasing Muscle Mass

Nutrient	Amount each day (in g per kg of body weight)
Protein	1.5–1.7 for muscle growth in men 1.3–1.5 for muscle growth in women 1.0–1.2 to maintain muscle mass in men and women
Carbohydrate	4–5 for 30–60 minute workout/day 6–8 for 60–90 minute workout/day
Fat	0.6–1.0
Possible supplements	Creatine (see chapter 8) Sports drinks (see chapter 5) Hydroxy methylbutyrate (see chapter 8)

supplement is not necessarily being converted to muscle—it's being converted to muscle fuel (glucose), allowing a longer workout, which in turn is increasing muscle mass, just as carbohydrate would have done.

Although you might hear that you need to eat 30 grams of protein after a workout, the truth is that we don't know how much protein athletes need, the best type of protein, or the best time to eat it after a workout, although we have a good idea as to how much protein they need over 24 hours. If you eat 1.5 to 1.7 grams of protein per kilogram of body weight per day (men) or 1.3 to 1.5 grams per kilogram of body weight per day (women) early in a weight training program, you will be getting enough protein for muscle growth. That's about 120 to 135 grams of protein for an 80-kilogram (176-lb) man, or 85 to 100 grams of protein for a 65-kilogram (143-lb) woman. This can be readily achieved by eating a normal diet.

Eat Plenty of Carbohydrate

Muscles get bigger and stronger with resistance training, such as weight training. It makes sense to feed the muscles high-carbohydrate food so they have the fuel to get them through a tough training session. You will need a minimum of 4 grams of carbohydrate per kilogram of body weight to fuel a workout; more if your training is heavy or intense. The trick is to eat extra good-quality food to fuel both the workout and the gain in muscle mass, without putting on extra weight as fat. That might mean an extra 2,100 to 4,200 kilojoules (500 to 1,000 cal) a day.

There is good evidence that eating a mix of protein and carbohydrate before and after a workout could well help promote muscle repair or, at least, minimise muscle breakdown after exercise. Having an adequate amount of carbohydrate before a workout will make you less likely to use muscle protein as a fuel, and eating a mix of protein and carbohydrate after training reduces the amount of muscle breakdown. A snack or meal with both protein and carbohydrate also promotes muscle protein synthesis. The carbohydrate stimulates insulin production, and the insulin helps protein uptake by the muscles. It is not clear what may be the best mix of protein and carbohydrate, but the evidence suggests that the meals need to be more carbohydrate than protein, meaning that flavoured milk, bread, rice, pasta, granola bars and muesli bars can be part of the ideal muscle building diet. (See chapter 7 for more advice on what to eat after sport.)

To summarise the previous two points, "A moderate level of carbohydrate should be ingested to maintain workout intensity and an adequate protein intake will help prevent muscle mass loss" (Lambert, Frank and Evans 2004, p. 325).

Eat Frequently

Athletes need to eat frequently, especially if they are doing a lot of training. That means three meals and three or more snacks a day. If you eat too little, you will not have enough fuel to train efficiently. Some people like to follow a set plan; for example, eating every two hours. It's up to you. I think you can be less regimented and still achieve your goals.

Don't skimp on an eating opportunity. Eat something before going to bed. Supper provides an extra nutrition boost and is useful for topping up your glycogen stores before an early-morning training session. If it's high in carbohydrate and low in fat, and you are an active person, it won't turn to body fat.

Concentrate the Kilojoules

Without enough kilojoules, your body won't have the means to create extra muscle mass. One very effective way of getting more nutrition is to make your meals and snacks energy dense; that is, more concentrated in kilojoules. This is an important technique for the athlete who is unintentionally losing weight or having difficulty gaining weight. Eating more food may not be a practical option. By fitting more kilojoules into the same amount of food, you don't end up eating a mountain of food. There are simple ways of getting more nutrition into food (e.g., adding nonfat milk powder and table margarine to a mashed potato).

Try some extra nutritious foods that are high in carbohydrate and low in fat but simple to eat in addition to your normal meals. Aim to get another 100+ grams of carbohydrate into your diet to support the energy needs of your training program and encourage weight gain. You could possibly fit in more bread, rice, pasta, flavoured yogurt, breakfast cereal, dried fruit, fruit juice, flavoured milk or food bars (see table 11.2). For extra kilojoules with healthy fat, eat more nuts, peanut butter, avocado, olive oil and other unsaturated oils.

Table 11.2 Examples of Nutritious, Energy-Dense Foods

Food	kJ/serve	cal/serve
Dried fruit, 1/2 cup	528	125
Nuts, 25 g (0.9 oz)	600	143
Peanut butter, 1 Tbsp	720	170
Avocado, 1/2 medium	1000	238
Unsaturated margarine, 1 Tbsp	600	143
Milo, Ovaltine, 2 Tbsp in 200 mL (7 oz) reduced-fat milk	760	180
Milk chocolate, 50 g (1.8 oz)	1040	248
Muesli bar, 1	500	120

Drink Plenty of Nutritious Fluids

Fluids provide a simple way of getting extra kilojoules. Drinks such as reduced-fat milk, milkshakes and smoothies (preferably made with reduced-fat milk or soy drinks) are very nutritious. You can add extra nonfat milk powder to milk for extra carbohydrate and protein. Commercial liquid meals such as Sustagen Sport are usually based on milk powder. You might also try plain fruit juices or add some yogurt to the juice.

Many protein supplemental drinks are on the market. Although many of them are nutritious, they are usually expensive. You can make your own at a fraction of the cost. Try some of the great Body Boost drink ideas below or make up the protein powder recipe (Glennergy) in chapter 2. I've named the first one Glenn's Gargantuan Gainer tongue in cheek, as many commercial products use titles to suggest rapid and massive muscle gain. Of course, muscle gains are slow and gradual.

Body Boost Drinks

Use these drinks to supplement your regular well-chosen diet. They are simple to make and inexpensive, and they provide a good balance of protein and carbohydrate without excess fat. They are ideal after a workout to replenish glycogen and stimulate muscle repair. Each recipe makes one serve.

Triple G (Glenn's Gargantuan Gainer)

Ingredients

250 mL (8 oz) nonfat or reduced-fat milk

3 Tbsp nonfat milk powder (30 g)

1 scoop ice cream

2 tsp Milo, Aktavite, Ovaltine, Nesquik or Horlicks

Method

Blend all ingredients together until smooth.

Nutrition Analysis

kJ:1425 (340 cal)

Fat: 7 g

Protein: 26 g

Carbohydrate: 47 g

Calcium: 880 mg

Iron: 2.5 mg

(continued)

Banana Powershake

Ingredients

250 mL (8 oz) nonfat or
reduced-fat milk
1 banana
1 scoop ice cream
1.5 Tbsp glucose powder or sugar
pinch nutmeg

Method

Blend first four ingredients together
until smooth. Sprinkle nutmeg on top.
Serve chilled.

Nutrition Analysis

kJ: 1715–1820 (410-435 cal)   Protein: 14 g   Calcium: 430 mg
Fat: 6 g (nonfat milk)   Carbohydrate: 75 g   Iron: negligible

Fruit Surge

Ingredients

250 mL (8 oz) nonfat or
reduced-fat milk
1 cup canned fruit
3 Tbsp nonfat milk powder (30 g)
1 scoop ice cream
1 Tbsp glucose powder or sugar

Method

Blend all ingredients and serve.

Nutrition Analysis

kJ: 1885–1990 (450-475 cal)   Protein: 26 g   Calcium: 850 mg
Fat: 5.5 g (nonfat milk)   Carbohydrate: 76 g   Iron: 1.0 mg

Sustagogo

Ingredients

200 mL (7 oz) reduced-fat milk
3 Tbsp Sustagen Sport powder

Method

Blend together and serve hot or cold.

Nutrition Analysis

kJ: 920 (220 cal)   Protein: 16 g   Calcium: 500 mg
Fat: 4 g   Carbohydrate: 32 g   Iron: 3.1 mg

Yojuice

Ingredients

200 mL (7 oz) fruit juice
3 Tbsp low-fat flavoured yogurt

Method

Blend ingredients and serve cold.

Nutrition Analysis

kJ: 500 (120 cal)   Protein: 4.2 g   Calcium: 120 mg
Fat: 0.2 g   Carbohydrate: 25 g   Iron: 0 mg

Avoid Most Nutritional Supplements

Many nutritional supplements are promoted as enhancing muscle growth. Unfortunately, the scientific studies do not justify the hype surrounding many of these supplements. I will briefly describe the supplements that may be of some value for increasing muscle. For more detail on each one, see chapter 8.

The early research suggests that the nonessential amino acid glutamine may assist in muscle growth in athletes involved in intense exercise, but far more research is required before we can promote its use. Adequate protein intake is likely to cover the body's need for glutamine.

Creatine certainly increases weight gain in many athletes, with an initial gain in the region of 1 to 3 kilograms (2 to 6 lb). What proportion of that weight gain is muscle mass and what is fluid retention is under dispute. Any sustained weight gain is likely to be extra muscle mass providing you are also doing a regular weight training program. Creatine allows you to do extra repetitions, leading to muscle growth.

Hydroxy methylbutyrate (HMB) studies suggest that it can reduce muscle damage during resistance exercise and help increase muscle mass. Any benefit is most likely to be in elite athletes and serious recreational athletes because they usually work their muscles hard. Fitness enthusiasts may get little benefit as they usually suffer less muscle damage after exercise.

Other supplements, such as chromium picolinate, vanadyl sulphate and boron, do not seem to provide any benefit to weight training athletes in either muscle strength or muscle mass.

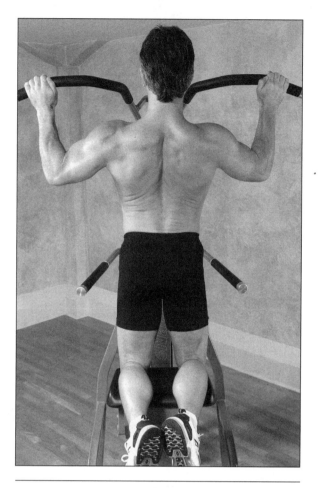

Adequate carbohydrate and protein are the key nutrients to increasing muscle growth when weight training.

Cutting Up

In the month before competition, bodybuilders go through the process of 'cutting up' to enhance muscle definition. They consume a very low fat diet to reduce subcutaneous fat. Bodybuilders who dramatically restrict their food intake before competition run the risk of losing muscle mass. That's because when there

Can Muscle Turn to Fat?

No, not if you mean a direct conversion from one to the other. If you don't use a muscle group, it will get smaller (atrophy). If, at the same time, your exercise levels drop or you start eating too much food, then the excess kilojoules will be stored as body fat.

The extra muscle produced by resistance training is great for weight control. Extra muscle needs extra kilojoules to maintain the increased metabolic rate. Extra kilojoules burned are kilojoules *not* stored as body fat.

is too little food, the body breaks down muscle for fuel. That makes all the hard work in the gym a waste. Ensure that you consume enough carbohydrate to spare your muscle stores from degradation.

Some believe that carbohydrate loading can increase muscle girth. For every extra gram of glycogen stored, an extra 2.4 to 4.0 grams of water are stored, which is believed to plump up the muscle size. However, one well-controlled study was unable to find any muscle definition difference between bodybuilders who carbohydrate-loaded and those who ate a regular diet before competition (Balon, Horowitz and Fitzsimmons 1992).

Some bodybuilders will dehydrate in the 24 hours before competition as this may make the skin 'tighter' to improve muscle definition. Unfortunately, dehydration can cause fatigue, headaches and faintness, which is not the best way to feel just before the competition starts. 'Fat mobilisers' are also popular during the cutting-up phase, even though they do not help with loss of body fat at all. Read the section on fat mobilisers in chapter 8. It could save you a pile of money.

FINAL SCORE

- Increasing muscle mass requires a combination of the right genes, resistance training, good nutrition and patience.
- Nutrition for increasing muscle mass comprises adequate carbohydrate for training and adequate protein and kilojoules for muscle growth.
- You will likely need 5 to 6 grams of carbohydrate per kilogram of body weight each day to fuel weight training workouts. It is also likely that you will need around 1.5 grams of protein per kilogram of body weight daily while you are increasing muscle mass.
- Eat a meal or snack with a mix of protein and carbohydrate soon after a workout to help replenish muscle glycogen stores and repair muscle protein damage.
- Many nutritional supplements promoting muscle growth are not well researched, or the research suggests little or no value. Creatine and HMB are two supplements that may assist muscle growth in those doing adequate resistance exercise.

twelve

Fat Burning and Weight Loss Strategies

Laffit Pincay Junior, 54, is a jockey of legendary status in U.S. racing. In a career encompassing over 35 years he has ridden over 9,200 winners, the most of any rider. A story is told of Pincay, who, while on a plane flight, took a single peanut from the packet, broke it in half and ate the first portion, saving the second half to eat later in the flight!

B e assured, you will not have to go to the lengths Laffit Pincay went to lose excess body fat. Active people are normally lean, but plenty of fit people still have difficulty shedding very small amounts of weight. This chapter details the best eating strategy for long-term success in losing body fat, or not gaining any, and keeping lean. If you are looking for a quick fix, a magic diet or a rapid weight loss program, you will not find it here because they rarely work and are generally unhealthy. They work only for as long as you can handle plain starvation.

Questions Athletes Ask

If you are carrying a little too much body fat, then your first step is to set yourself a realistic goal. Your goal may not even be a set weight. Your goal could rightfully be just to feel a lot better and fitter than you do now. Be warned, before you go any further, that this is not a food-obsessed chapter that will ask you to measure everything you eat and delete every taste pleasure you ever pursued. If you want that, buy the latest diet book. This chapter is about eating to successfully control your weight while including such foods as wine, chocolate, pizza or ice cream on occasion. Successful people don't 'diet'. Success depends more on what goes on inside your head than on what goes on your plate. That is, your attitude will determine your success. Let me answer four common questions before I explain further.

Why Do I Put on Body Fat?

Please appreciate that you are designed to gain body fat. Humans evolved to gain body fat easily when food was abundant, as that extra stored body fat acted as an energy reserve during food shortages. Those that put on body fat easily were better able to survive the rigours of human survival. If you gain body fat easily,

The Shane Warne Weight Loss Program

'No pizzas, toasted cheese sandwiches, hot chips, potato chips, sausage rolls, vanilla slices—there's not much left for me except for cereal and some baked beans', revealed cricketer Shane Warne in a 2002 press briefing during a tour in South Africa. 'I haven't eaten pizzas or drunk beers for the last couple of weeks. I've dropped about eight kilos'.

you are normal. If it is difficult to lose body fat, you are normal. To lose body fat, or not gain it, you must treat your body as it was designed. That often means eating more vegetables and fruit, eating less treat foods and doing more activity even if you are already fit.

As you age, your body weight will tend to increase. One contributing factor is that your metabolic rate decreases with age, but the more common reason is that we do less activity as we age without eating less food. Regular exercise and weight training to increase muscle mass will keep your metabolic rate elevated and slow any age-related weight gain.

Am I Too Fat?

Scientists use all types of formulas to judge whether someone is too fat. I think the easiest numbers to remember are 90 and 100. They refer to the perimeter of your waist in centimetres, with 90 centimetres (35 in.) being the maximum for women and 100 centimetres (39 in.) being the maximum for men. The measurement should be done in line with the belly button for men and at the narrowest part of the waist, just above the hips, for women.

Why measure here? Because it is the fat around your middle that is the most dangerous to your health. Once that gets above the recommended circumference, your health can decline. Fat here will raise blood cholesterol and blood pressure, while dramatically increasing your risk of diabetes. Get a tape measure and find the circumference of your middle (see figure 12.1). If you are overfat, change your eating and exercise habits such that your belt goes in a notch every few weeks or so. If your waist is normal, then eat sensibly and remain active to ensure that it stays that way.

What Causes Athletes to Gain Weight?

- **Off-season.** Less training and more time for partying can be a simple recipe for gaining extra body fat. This is common in athletes involved in team sports that often have a two-month break after the season has ended.

- **Injury.** Again, a lower training level is the key reason for weight gain. Being injured can also mean feeling depressed because you can't compete, possibly turning you to food for solace. A sports psychologist can help you with your thinking.

- **Alcohol.** Alcoholic drinks are strongly associated with male team sports. Alcohol is also strongly associated with dehydration, poor sports performance, poor recovery from injury, and increases in body fat. Alcohol needs to be treated with respect.

- **Grease.** Too much fat in foods, and a reliance on take-away foods, can easily make your navel move farther from your spine. Choosing less energy-dense foods and drinks will help control body weight.

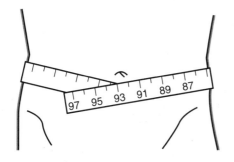

Figure 12.1 Waist measurement (at the level of the belly button) should be less than 90 centimetres (35 in.) for women and 100 centimetres (39 in.) for men. More than this can contribute to poor health due to being overweight.

You can also determine your body mass index (BMI), a common indicator of 'fatness' based on your height and weight using the following equation:

$$BMI = Weight \ (kg) \div Height \ (m)^2$$

For example, if you weigh 80 kilograms (176 lb) and you are 180 centimetres (1.8 m; 5 ft 11 in.) tall, then your BMI is 24.7:

$$\frac{80}{1.8 \times 1.8} = 80 \div 3.24 = 24.7$$

A BMI between 20 and 25 is considered a healthy weight. A person with a BMI over 25 is considered overweight, whereas someone with a BMI over 30 is considered obese. The BMI is not always the best measurement of overweight in athletes because it doesn't account for muscle mass. A well-muscled athlete is likely to have a BMI higher than 25, yet can still have a low body fat level. In these circumstances, your waist measurement is a better gauge of 'fatness'.

A common way to determine the fat levels of athletes is to measure their skinfolds. This should be done by a trained kinanthropometrist using a set of skinfold callipers to determine the levels of body fat just below the skin. Various sites can be measured, with the most common being the biceps, triceps, subscapula (just beneath the shoulder blade) and abdomen (just beneath the rib cage). A sum of the measurements gives an indication of the level of 'fatness'. The same person should do the measurements with the same callipers on the same sites to ensure consistency. The measurements are commonly done on elite athletes to find the measurements that provide the best performance. Recreational athletes probably need no more than a waist measurement to determine a good level of body fat for their best performance.

Please be aware that not all athletes want to be superlean. Obviously, some sports require bulk rather than speed, in which case a little extra body fat is acceptable. Yes, sumo wrestlers are an obvious example, but consider long-distance open-water swimmers. They often swim in cold waters, and extra body fat provides insulation against the cold as well as some buoyancy.

Can I Lose Weight Fast?

The answer is no. Well, not if you want to remain healthy and sane. It is easy to believe that we have become fat really fast and that Christmas, Easter or the annual holiday is to blame for the excess weight. This is very unlikely. Most athletes will gain weight slowly and gradually over a period of months. During a layoff as a result of injury or the end-of-season break, an athlete could gain 2 to 5 kilograms (4 to 11 lb). This process needs to be reversed

The Cathy Freeman 'If Shane Can Do It, So Can I' Weight Loss Program

'Fruit, vegetables, water, skin off the chicken, no McDonalds, no alcohol—oh, maybe one or two glasses of red wine—but training hard is the thing', is the secret of Cathy Freeman, 400-metre Olympic gold medalist, Sydney 2000. In 2002 she had gone from 65 kilograms (143 lb) to 54 kilograms (119 lb) in ten weeks. 'It's no big deal', she said as she closed in on her 52-kilogram (114-lb) 'fighting weight'.

gradually and permanently, ideally at a rate of 0.5 kilograms (1 lb) per week . It may sound frustratingly slow, but a faster rate could result in a loss of muscle.

Some simple changes to your diet could be all that is required. For example, if you changed from drinking 600 mL (20 oz) of full-cream milk a day to a reduced-fat milk, you would save 150,000 kilojoules (35,800 cal) a year. Potentially, that's a loss of 5 kilograms (11 lb) per year. Instead of two cream biscuits for morning tea, eat a piece of fruit to save well over 200,000 kilojoules (47,800 cal) a year, a potential loss of 6.5 kilograms (14 lb). Simple changes to your eating can make a big difference—over time.

If you are a jockey, boxer, lightweight rower, bodybuilder, wrestler, diver, figure skater or gymnast, you are probably under pressure to be a certain weight or shape. Being 2 or 3 kilos over your 'fighting weight' can come as a shock, so you want to get it off fast.

The first problem with this issue is the term *fast*. *Fast* means that you will have to do just that: fast . . . as in 'go without food'. Without food, or following a very restricted diet, your body runs out of glycogen and dumps the water needed to store that glycogen. In other words, you run out of energy and lose weight mainly as water.

Rapid weight loss, especially by dehydration, will torpedo your endurance as well as your sprinting or intense training programs. Rapid weight loss can also affect your thinking and concentration—feeling tired and irritable is not the best way to go into an event.

You may need to ask yourself, Am I competing in the right weight class for my natural weight and health? There is little point in becoming weak and wasted just to make a lower weight class. A thin athlete is not always a fast athlete, and a hungry athlete is a weak athlete. You would be smart to plan weeks, not days, ahead and get those extra kilos off slowly and permanently. That way you retain your health, strength and ability, both physical and mental.

How Can I Raise My Metabolism?

You may already know that your basal metabolic rate (BMR) burns quite a few kilojoules each day. Your BMR is the energy burned to keep you alive—that is, to keep your heart beating; lungs breathing; and liver, kidneys

and brain functioning. You can estimate your BMR using the following equations:

Male

$$15 \times \text{body weight (kg)} + 716 = \text{cal}$$

$$(63 \times \text{body weight [kg]} + 3,000 = \text{kJ})$$

Female

$$12 \times \text{body weight (kg)} + 716 = \text{cal}$$

$$(50 \times \text{body weight [kg]} + 3,000 = \text{kJ})$$

Adjustments for Age

30–35 yr	reduce BMR by 5%
36–50 yr	reduce BMR by 10%
51–69 yr	reduce BMR by 15%
70+ yr	reduce BMR by 20%

Reprinted from *Nutrition research*, Vol. 19, A. Movahedi, "Simple formula for calculating basal energy expenditure," pp. 989-995, Copyright 1999, with permission from Elsevier.

When you do the calculations, there is a good chance you will have a figure of 5,000 to 6,700 kilojoules (1,200 to 1,600 cal) for women and 5,800 to 8,400 kilojoules (1,400 to 2,000 cal) for men. For example, if you are a 32-year-old 65-kilogram (143-lb) woman, your BMR will be about 6,250 kilojoules (50 × 65, then add 3,000, then take off 5%) or 1,420 calories. A healthy adult is very unlikely to have a BMR less than 4,200 kilojoules (1,000 cal), when measured accurately.

A common question is, How can I raise my metabolism? People hope to be able to help the body burn fat while they are at their desks or sleeping. The answer is, Yes, you can raise your metabolism, but there is not an easy method. The three most effective ways to raise your basal metabolic rate are as follows:

• **Exercise.** This is by far the best method. Exercise burns kilojoules and generally increases your muscle mass depending on the exercise. Swimming will increase upper body muscle, and running will increase lower body muscle. I suspect that you already have this method as part of your life.

• **Weight training.** Muscles have a higher metabolic rate than body fat has. Weight training is the most effective way of increasing muscle mass, but don't rely on it as the sole method of losing body fat. Aerobic exercise will usually burn up fat stores at a faster rate. You could, of course, do light weights as part of a general fitness program.

The Lauren Burns Weight Loss Program

For the 2000 Sydney Olympics, the taekwondo gold medalist Lauren Burns had to work hard to compete in the under-49-kilogram division. 'It took me three months, because under 49 kg is way too light for me. I had the help of the Victorian Institute of Sport and its dietitians', said Lauren, who now weighs 54 kilograms. 'That's my natural weight', she said.

- **Small, frequent meals.** Some research has suggested that dividing your food into five or six smaller meals helps raise metabolic rate compared to eating just one or two big meals in the day.

Often, you will hear stories that certain foods will raise your metabolic rate above what it is normally. You may hear, for example, that chilli, green tea and caffeine raise metabolic rate. This is true, but it is unlikely that you can eat enough chilli or drink enough cups of green tea at every meal, day after day, to make a big difference to your metabolic rate. You might burn an extra 200 kilojoules (50 cal) per day, but that doesn't hold a candle to the 1,250 kilojoules (300 cal) burned in a 45-minute walk or the 820 kilojoules (200 cal) saved by cutting out the two cream biscuits at coffee break.

Body Shape

There is a great deal of pressure to conform to cultural ideals of the ideal body shape. Providing that your waist circumference is within the guides given earlier in the chapter, then your shape may not be easy to change. Compare the body shapes of the athletes in figure 12.2. They are all lean athletes, but they have different body shapes. Sure, exercise or weight training will improve your musculature, but beyond that you are better off accepting your shape than trying mythical ways to sculpt your body to some ideal shape. For example, it is well established that you cannot 'spot' reduce. Doing abdominal exercises will improve

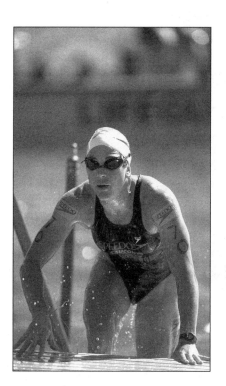
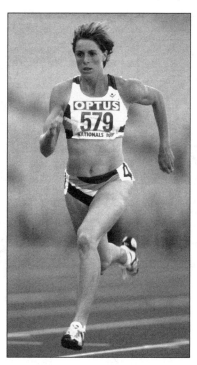
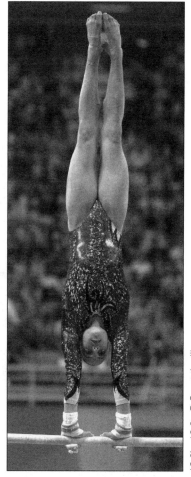

Figure 12.2   Lean bodies can come in a variety of shapes.

the strength of the abdominal muscles, but it won't magically get rid of abdominal fat. The only way you can do that is to eat less energy than you burn.

> It is an amazing paradox that our culture, with its great flexibility and liberal ideas, attempts to superimpose one form of body build on those whom nature has endowed differently.
>
> *Hilda Bruch (1957)*

If your waist circumference does not fall within the guides given earlier in this chapter, then you may want to evaluate whether your body shape is normal and healthy. The pear body shape is generally a female shape with fat deposits on the hips, thighs and buttocks (see figure 12.3). This is normal for women. Human survival relied on women having fat in this part of the body so that, if there was a food shortage, they had fat reserves to ensure that pregnancies went to term and that they could also breastfeed the infant. As the Western diet hasn't had a food shortage in the last 50 years, we haven't had to rely on fat stores for survival.

The apple shape is associated with excess body fat in men and women. Excess body fat around the abdomen is a long-term health risk as it can raise blood cholesterol, blood pressure and blood glucose levels, leading to a higher risk of heart disease, stroke and diabetes. Apple-shaped people also have a greater chance of back pain and breast and bowel cancer. In short, pear shape = healthy, apple shape = unhealthy, although no one should gain excess weight, no matter their shape.

Fad Products

Before you think about changing your food choices, you will first need to ignore the distractions of weight loss charlatans promoting fad diets and slimming products. History has taught us that there has never been a 'weight loss breakthrough'. It is reasonable to suggest that there is unlikely to be a healthy, simple new idea or product that will make body fat loss easy. You can buy diet books, products (fat metabolisers, tablets, meal replacement drinks), weight loss machinery, diet soaps, diet soups or cellulite tablets, but all these will prove disappointing as you are really buying hope, not success. Why don't they work? Let's take a brief look at some of them.

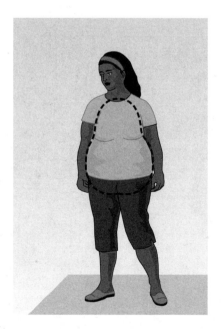
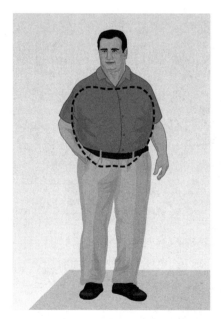

Figure 12.3 The pear shape is commonly found in women and is not linked to any health problems. The apple shape occurs when abdominal fat increases, which in turn increases the chance of heart disease, diabetes and other medical problems.

Reprinted, by permission, from J.H. Wilmore and D.L. Costill, 2004, *Physiology of sport and exercise*, 3rd ed. (Champaign, IL: Human Kinetics), 679.

Diet Books

Every diet book is written to a formula. They are all prescriptive and restrictive. That is, they dictate what you eat and they cut out a huge range of foods, including all your favourite foods. If you don't follow their exact program, you probably won't lose weight. For a diet book to work, it must control your actions and decisions. Take a diet book, any diet book, and this is what you will be told:

- You can't eat pastries, take-aways, snack food, soft drinks, confectionery (candy), biscuits, cakes, fatty foods, butter and margarine or any treat you might enjoy.
- You can eat vegetables, legumes, lean meats, low-fat dairy foods, fruits and whole-grain cereals (unless it is a low-carbohydrate book in which cereals and some fruits are deleted).

Over the years, the low-carbohydrate diet has been promoted to athletes and the public alike. It is interesting to note that low-carbohydrate diets have been popular since the 1950s. (The first one was published by William Banting in 1864, over 140 years ago, so it is not a new idea.) In 2003 researchers from Stanford University checked all the research on low-carbohydrate diets and concluded that they only work because they are low-kilojoule diets (Bravata et al. 2003).

A low-carbohydrate diet book often mentions that you can eat all the fat you like. That sounds great until you realise that there aren't any potatoes for the sour cream, no bread for the butter, no pasta or rice for the oil, no fruit for the cream. Ever tried eating fat on its own? Of course not. By deleting the carbohydrate, you also end up eating less fat and therefore fewer kilojoules.

When you limit food intake to low-carbohydrate foods such as salad vegetables, lean meats, cheese, yogurt and a small number of fruits, it becomes very difficult to overeat. Of course, when you limit food to fruits, vegetables, oats, pasta, rice, bread, lean meats, low-fat dairy foods and the occasional treat, it is also difficult to overeat. The latter style is called healthy eating, a concept too difficult to embrace by pop nutritionists.

Do low-carbohydrate diets work? Yes, in the short term; no, in the long term. The low-carbohydrate diet can produce greater weight loss over three to six months, but there is little difference between low-carbohydrate eating and low-kilojoule eating after 12 months. It is also important to note that there is a very high drop-out level for both types of diets, which should remind us all that any weight loss diet is hard to stick to.

If foods high in carbohydrate were implicated in weight gain, why have we conveniently forgotten the Pritikin Diet, the wonder diet of the 1970s and 1980s? It was a very high carbohydrate, low-fat diet that trimmed the body fat off millions. Clearly, carbohydrate wasn't fattening itself. The Pritikin Diet was so extreme in its avoidance of fat that most people returned to their old style of eating very quickly and replaced any lost weight.

All the emphasis on reducing carbohydrate has forgotten that athletes and other active people need carbohydrate for muscle fuel. Depriving endurance athletes of their carbohydrate will reduce their endurance capacity. As a result, they will tire quickly and not meet their performance goals.

I agree with the 2005 Dietary Guidelines for Americans, which states:

> When it comes to body weight control, it is calories that count—not the proportions of fat, carbohydrates, and protein in the diet. Diets that provide very low or very high amounts of protein, carbohydrates, or fat are likely to provide low amounts of some nutrients and are not advisable for long-term use. Although these kinds of weight-loss diets have been shown to result in weight reduction, the maintenance of a reduced weight ultimately will depend on a change in lifestyle.

Magic Products

Fat 'metabolisers' or 'mobilisers' are touted as weight loss agents, especially to bodybuilders and personal trainers. Common claims are that they 'convert fat to body fuel' and 'improve muscle definition', making them attractive to anyone trying to lose body fat. The brochures imply that they will melt away the excess fat, turning you into 'chiselled' beefcake or beach babe in no time. However, they only work 'in conjunction with a calorie-controlled diet', which is their way of saying, 'if you want to lose weight, eat less kilojoules, but please buy our supplement so you get the impression the supplement also played a role'.

The most common ingredients of fat metabolisers are the compounds carnitine, inositol and choline. Other ingredients might be lecithin, methionine, herbs and vitamins. There is no scientific evidence that any of these ingredients cause fat loss or help to control your appetite.

Another favourite claim is that certain products stop you from digesting fat or carbohydrate. The fact is that undigested fat or carbohydrate would pass into your large intestine, causing abdominal pain, gas and diarrhea. The manufacturer of the product chitosan claimed that it binds to fat in the gut and passes undigested into the stool. In 2003, University of California researchers revealed that a full daily dose of chitosan saved 42 kilojoules (10 cal), the amount of energy burned in a two-minute walk (Gades and Stern 2003)! Other research shows that chitosan did not assist in the loss of body fat (Ni Mhurchu et al. 2004). (Chitosan is not to be confused with the drug Xenical, which does reduce fat digestion and absorption, but you have to be on a low-fat diet in the first place so that you don't get diarrhea. Xenical is available from chemists.)

Some products are plain ridiculous, such as slimming soap, which supposedly dissolves fat from your thighs and waist as you wash. This is a rip-off at the criminal end of the scale. Yes, people do buy this stuff . . . but only once. In summary, don't waste your time or money on weight loss diets or gimmicks. To lose excess body fat, you must eat less energy (kilojoules or calories) than you burn up each day. Why? Because that is the first law of thermodynamics—it's been in place since the beginning of time. To lose excess body fat, you must be prepared to do extra training, or modify your eating, which is discussed later in this chapter.

The Facts About Cellulite

Even if you are fit and eat well, and your waist measurement is normal, you may still have cellulite. What is cellulite? According to *Taber's Cyclopedic Medical Dictionary* (19th edition), cellulite is a 'non-technical term for subcutaneous deposits of fat, especially in the buttocks, legs and thighs' (p. 372). Put simply, cellulite is round, fatty lumps just under the skin and features mainly in women. Having cellulite doesn't mean you have excess fat.

'Cellulite' fat stores and regular fat stores appear to differ structurally. In cellulite, fibrous connective tissue separates the fat cells into clusters (see figure 12.4). Much of the connective tissue is collagen, a protein. With age, extra collagen is formed to change the structural geography of the stored fat. Evidence suggests that blood flow in the cellulitic areas is slower, but the role this plays is unclear.

These changes encourage a mild edema in the area, with the extra water giving rise to the orange peel look. Further pronouncement of the cellulite occurs if the fat cells enlarge and the skin loses elasticity with time. Certainly, a greater amount of fluid appears to be associated with cellulite areas when compared to other areas of body fat. One theory is that cellulite has a higher level of proteoglycans, molecules of proteins and sugars combined, which have high water-attracting properties.

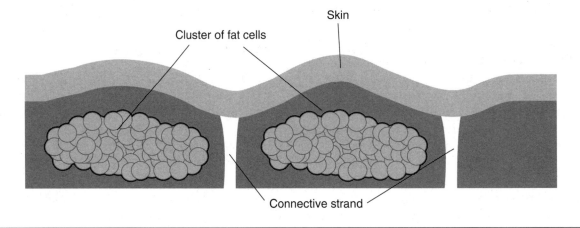

Figure 12.4 Cellulite consists of clusters of fat cells underneath the skin, giving the skin a dimpled appearance.

Cellulite often increases with age, possibly compounded by female sex hormones and extra weight. Cellulite is more common in white women than in black or Asian women.

The cellulite effect may become more obvious in the following cases:

- In overweight women as fat cells enlarge and the fat begins to bulge from the fat cell compartments. Fat cells can only enlarge to a certain size. If more fat needs to be stored, the body must produce new fat cells.

- With high-salt diets as the sodium may cause more fluid retention. Just deleting salt at the dinner table may not help as about 80 per cent of all salt in the diet is added by food manufacturers. A better choice is to eat reduced-salt foods.

- During the week premenses with fluid retention.

Unfortunately, once a fat cell has been created, it stays forever. It can be reduced in size, but it won't go away. Cellulite is more common in women because their skin is thinner and their fat compartments larger and more rounded than in men. The result is a dimpling appearance on the surface of the skin. It can occur in overweight and normal weight women. If a woman has cellulite, then her daughters are more likely to have cellulite. Genetics can be a nuisance sometimes.

Cellulite is not a buildup of toxic waste or undigested food, and it is not caused by faulty circulation as has been claimed in the past. Cellulite creams are not part of the solution. The creams seemed to work because gentle massaging of the skin will temporarily flatten some of the bumpy areas. In other words, you can rub whatever you like into the 'cellulite' area and the skin will become smoother for a short time.

Wise Food Choices

No matter how you look at it, gaining body fat is due to eating more kilojoules than you burn through activity each day. This may be only a small discrepancy, with an average body fat gain of 1 to 3 grams a day (30 to 90 kJ [7 to 21 cal]) a day. That's around 1 to 3 kilograms (2.2 to 6.6 lb) every three years. (Note: Although food fat is 37 kJ [9 cal] per gram, body fat is 29 kJ [7 cal] per gram as some water is integrated with body fat.)

Fat loss is the opposite: You need to eat fewer kilojoules than you use each day so that you are forced to burn a little extra body fat each day. For some athletes, this is not easy. You may not succeed the first time around. Don't despair. This may take more than one attempt. Indeed, most successful people will tell you that they made more than one attempt to achieve their fat loss goals. A few food tricks can help put the odds in your favour, but don't for a moment expect this to be easy.

In 1980, Coca-Cola began to design a new diet drink. The can itself went through 150 designs, and over 10,000 consumers had taste-tested Diet Coke before its release in July 1982 using saccharin as the sweetener. By the end of 1983, Diet Coke was sweetened with the intense sweeteners saccharin and aspartame, before it eventually dispensed with saccharin (which, by the way, was cleared of all links with human cancer in May 2000). Unfortunately, the whole concept of sugar substitutes gave the impression that sugar was fattening and that the elimination of sugar was the road to salvation. Not so. Let me explain some nutrition points and link them to weight loss.

First, we must understand the origin of energy (kilojoules and calories). Only four

The Dean Lukin 'Yeah, Did That Years Ago' Weight Loss Program

Los Angeles Olympics gold medal super-heavyweight weightlifter, Dean Lukin, went from 145 kilograms (319 lb) in 1984 to a lean 95 kilograms (209 lb) eight years later. He revealed all in *The Dean Lukin Diet* In the book he described being a big lad and going to his girlfriend's house for dinner. He sat on the toilet and crushed the porcelain bowl, breaking it into jagged pieces. 'I have never been so thankful for the invention of toilet seats', said Lukin. Dean does hand out lots of sensible nutrition advice in the book. Guess that's why it wasn't a best-seller.

Table 12.1 Energy Value of Food Components

Food component	Kilojoules per gram	Calories per gram
Protein	17	4
Fat	37	9
Carbohydrate	16	4
Alcohol	29	7

components of the diet contribute energy: protein, fat, carbohydrate and alcohol. Fat and alcohol, when compared gram for gram, have around twice the kilojoules as protein or carbohydrate (see table 12.1). Therefore, it makes sense to limit the amount of fat and alcohol you consume if you want to lose excess body fat. Indeed, the scientific evidence supports this as the best decision.

Eat for Fat Loss

The dietary basics to lose body fat are to eat less fat and alcohol, and possibly eat more carbohydrate foods. This is the current, universally accepted style of eating for health and shedding body fat. Most adults gain weight because they eat too much fat, too much alcohol and not enough staple foods such as fruits, vegetables and cereals.

It is now well established that the fat in food is quite easy to convert to body fat. If you eat an extra 100 fat kilojoules, 97 of them will go straight onto your waist. Carbohydrate and excess protein are generally used for energy production and are unlikely to be converted to body fat. Here, it must be noted that carbohydrate foods include sugars and starches; there-

fore, sugar in modest amounts is unlikely to be fattening. Protein and carbohydrate intakes are tightly regulated, and any excess consumption is burned up by the body rather than being stored as fat, although there is evidence that fat people are capable of converting some carbohydrate to body fat.

The body will preferentially convert food carbohydrate to blood glucose and glycogen stored in muscle and in the liver. Glucose is your primary muscle and brain fuel. Without carbohydrate you will have to convert muscle or food proteins to glucose, because fat is very poorly and inefficiently converted to glucose. Although it is possible to eat excess carbohydrate, in real life this is difficult if those carbohydrate foods are fruits, vegetables and whole-grain cereals. It is rare to find anyone who eats 'too much' fruit and vegetables; indeed, 9 out of 10 adults eat too few.

Fat also has a poor feedback mechanism on appetite so it is easy to overconsume fatty foods before they satisfy the appetite. Both carbohydrate and protein are much more efficient at telling the body when it is full so they tend not to be overconsumed. Beyond this, there is good evidence that foods with a high water content have a strong ability to satisfy the appetite for a relatively few kilojoules. I have summarised the effects of the different food components on your appetite and their ability to become excess body fat in table 12.2.

In a series of experiments, University of Sydney researchers showed that different foods with equal amounts of kilojoules had widely differing abilities to satisfy the appetite (Holt et al. 1995). For example, for the same number of kilojoules, boiled potatoes were six times more filling than a croissant. The upshot of this work was that foods with a high water content and

Table 12.2 Influence of Different Food Components on Body Fat

Food component	Energy content	Effect on your satiety	Ability to convert excess to body fat	Ability to make you fat
Fat	High	Moderate	Easy	High
Protein	Low	Good	Hard	Poor
Carbohydrate	Low	Good	Hard	Poor
Alcohol	Moderate	Moderate	Hard	Moderate
Water	Nil	Good	Nil	Nil

a low fat content such as fruits and vegetables were far more satisfying than foods with a low water content and a high fat content such as cakes and pastries.

The University of Sydney study also revealed that high-protein, low-fat foods such as lean meat and fish had a high level of satiety (appetite suppression). You can see why a meal of meat and vegetables or salad is very satisfying. (Of course, this natural appetite-suppressing effect can be overridden at all-you-can-eat smorgasbord meals, Christmas dinner and other special events.)

We are conditioned to eat the same amount of food each day. I don't mean the same amount of kilojoules, but the same volume of food. Dr. Barbara Rolls' research at Pennsylvania State University, USA, revealed that we eat roughly the same weight or volume of food each day (Rolls and Bell 1999). Think about it. No matter what you do, you probably eat the same breakfast five or six days a week. You probably also expect the same amount of food on your dinner plate. If it is true that we eat the same volume of food each day, then it makes sense to eat foods with a low energy density—that is, low-fat, high-water, moderate-protein type foods (e.g., fruits and vegetables are around 90 per cent water and only 1 to 3 kJ per gram). Eating too much high-energy-density foods could be contributing to the midriff overhang. Table 12.3 shows the range of energy densities found in food.

Keep a Check on Fat

Fat is very energy dense; that is, it has a lot of kilojoules per gram compared to other food components. As table 12.1 shows, fat and alcohol have the most energy (in kilojoules or calories) per gram, making them the most energy dense components of food. This is why there is such a concern with the fat content of foods and why dietary fat has such a bad image.

I mentioned in chapter 1 that some diet advisers recommend that you count the fat in your diet, limiting it to 20 to 30 grams per day. That's a huge and dramatic drop when you consider that many people eat 80 to 100 grams of fat a day. Of course, if you want palatable and enjoyable meals, I suggest you don't go any lower than 40 grams per day for women, and 50 to 60 grams for men, who are active each day. Count fat grams if you wish, but don't become fat obsessed because the food may start

Table 12.3 Energy Density of Selected Foods

Food	Kilojoules per 100 g	Calories per 100 g
Mushroom	98	23
Apple	180	45
Banana	358	85
Potato, boiled	290	70
Milk, full cream	280	67
Milk, skim	146	35
Baked beans	395	90
Meat, lean	730	175
Bread	925	220
Muesli bar	1,680	400
Croissant	1,340	320
Meat pie	1,065	255
Potato crisps	2,100	500
Beer	170	40
Wine	315	75

to control you rather than vice versa. The most dangerous fat, of course, is saturated fats. You can use the Nutrient Food Value Chart at the end of the book to get an idea of the fat content of foods. Don't forget that some fat-containing foods such as the avocado, nuts, seeds and cheese are very nutritious and should still be able to find a place in your diet.

Drink Less Alcohol

Although small amounts of alcohol can protect against heart disease, they can also contribute to your waistline. Alcohol is dealt with as a toxic substance by the body so it must be metabolised preferentially ahead of other nutrients. As soon as the body absorbs alcohol, it starts to metabolise it at around 10 grams (one standard drink) each hour. Each gram of alcohol is 29 kilojoules (7 cal). If these kilojoules aren't burned up through activity, more food fat will be converted into body fat. Put another way, alcohol isn't converted to body fat, but it will 'push' more food fat into becoming body fat.

The figures for alcohol given in table 12.3 suggest that beer and wine are not very energy dense. Be aware, however, that most people

Fat, Carbohydrate and Protein

Following are some reasons for reducing fat intake:

- Fat is energy dense, having twice the kilojoules as carbohydrate or protein.
- Excess fat is easy to convert to body fat.
- Fat is less satisfying to the appetite compared to carbohydrate and protein. As a result, it is easier to overeat.
- Fatty foods (e.g., pastries, cakes, cookies) generally have low water content and a high energy density, which means they take longer to suppress the appetite. High-water-content foods seem to have a greater ability to satisfy the appetite than do high-fat, low-water foods.
- Keeping the fat, especially saturated fat, intake low may be the best nutrition strategy for long-term body fat loss and health.
- Many high-fat foods, such as crisps and snack foods, will also have a high salt content.

Following are benefits of eating more carbohydrate and having a moderate protein intake:

- Unrefined carbohydrate foods such as fruits, vegetables and legumes are very filling, making them difficult to overconsume.
- Lean protein foods such as lean meats and fish have a good ability to control appetite.
- Fruits, vegetables and legumes have a high water content, which makes them quite filling.
- High-carbohydrate and moderate-protein foods such as breads, cereals and legumes provide essential nutrients and fibre.
- Carbohydrate foods are your only source of fibre. Adequate fibre will keep you regular, whereas too little could clog your down-pipe.
- Fruits, vegetables, nuts, seeds and cereals are your major source of antioxidants, which are linked to a reduced risk of heart disease and cancer.
- Protein foods offer a range of minerals, with calcium (milk, yogurt, cheese), iron and zinc (meats) being the minerals of most importance.
- Adding some foods with 'natural' fat such as nuts, seeds, avocados and vegetable oils will enhance healthy eating, while still leaving some room for your favourite treats.

will easily drink much more beer and wine than, say, skim milk. Three cans of beer provide 1,890 kilojoules (450 cal), whereas a glass of skim milk provides 335 kilojoules (80 cal).

Can You Eat as Much Carbohydrate as You Like?

Carbohydrate is very efficiently stored as glycogen, but, on the rare occasion that liver and muscle glycogen stores are full, carbohydrate can be converted to body fat. Yet even when large amounts of carbohydrate are eaten, its conversion to fat is slow and inefficient. The body's major adaptation is to increase the amount of carbohydrate used as a fuel source and store any excess dietary fat as body fat. It is possible to eat too much carbohydrate (more than 800 g [28 oz] daily), but I have never seen a fit and healthy person eat carbohydrate to excess. Fat, yes; carbohydrate, no. Don't think that eating lots of cakes, biscuits and pastries is a carbohydrate problem. Most of their kilojoules come from fat. (Half the kilojoules in a cream biscuit come from fat.)

Following is an independent and unbiased view of the food and weight loss issue:

It is important to state that excess energy (Calories) in any form will promote body fat accumulation and that excess consumption of low fat foods, while not as obesity-producing as excess consumption of high fat foods, will lead to obesity if energy expenditure (exercise) is not increased.

That quote is the conclusion of the Joint FAO/WHO Expert Consultation (Food and Agriculture Organisation 1998). In other words, if you eat too much and exercise too little, you will become overweight.

A lower fat, higher carbohydrate diet is probably the best food balance to *minimise* body fat stores. This has been misinterpreted to mean that cutting out all sources of fat will make you thin. It won't if you continue to eat mountains of low-fat food and sit on your rear all day.

Successful and Permanent Weight Loss

As you are likely to be a fit and active person, then you are probably burning quite a few kilojoules each day. By focusing more on the energy consumed, you should achieve a steady rate of fat loss with some simple changes to your diet. I have given you what I think is the basis of successful fat loss. This is not just personal opinion. U.S. researchers have tracked 3,000 people who have lost at least 10 per cent of their body weight and kept that excess off for a year or more (Wing and Hill 2001). On average, the participants in this project lost 30 kilograms (66 lb) over five years. The researchers found that these successful weight maintainers had a lot in common. The most important factors in their success were as follows:

- They ate a healthy, low-fat diet (not a low-carbohydrate diet).
- They ate smaller portion sizes and rarely overate.
- They allowed themselves the occasional treat without concern.
- They exercised, or were active, for at least one hour each day.

- They kept tabs on their weight, but weren't obsessive about it. They quickly changed their food and exercise habits if their weight began to creep up.

The Relationship Between Food and Exercise

You have probably heard a few people say that exercise intensity and time of day are very important as to how much fat you burn up. Well, it doesn't really matter. The biggest factor for burning up body fat is whether you do the activity in the first place. It may be interesting to speculate whether you burn more fat in certain circumstances, but here is a general guide:

- To burn fat, you have to be active. The fitter you are, the better your body is at burning fat. To get a reasonable level of fitness, you need to get up and move your body for three to five hours a week.

- It doesn't really matter whether you exercise in the morning or afternoon, or whether you exercise before breakfast or after breakfast. People will tell you that you are a better 'fat burner' at certain times of the day, but this is without substantiation. If you exercise primarily for weight control, and your body burns more kilojoules than you consume in your diet, then you will be a 'fat burner', independent of when you exercise.

- It doesn't really matter whether you walk or jog. You will burn up more fat by jogging for 30 minutes than you will by walking for 30 minutes. On the other hand, you will burn up more fat by walking for 60 minutes than you will by jogging for 30 minutes.

- The amount of 'incidental activity' during the day will potentially burn more fat and kilojoules than a jog. Getting up from your chair, having a stretch or a quick walk around the office, taking the stairs up to the next floor, hand watering the garden and so on can burn more body fat through the day than a 30-minute walk. So, don't assume that 30 minutes of exercise a day is all you need to do for fat burning.

- For losing fat, weight-bearing exercises such as walking, aerobics and jogging are better at burning up fat stores than are weight-supported exercise such as swimming and cycling. However, it is better to do something you enjoy than to analyse its fat burning capabilities. Refer back to the first point.

Your Eating Habits

Sometimes, just the way people eat makes it very difficult to lose weight. Let me give you some examples.

• **Quick eaters.** Life is busy—so much to do, so little time. If you always eat your meals quickly, then you will likely eat more kilojoules than you need before your appetite is satisfied. Slow down your meals. Take time to chew your food. This will allow time for your body chemistry to assess when you have truly had enough to eat. The signal will come from a feeling of fullness.

• **Plate cleaners.** In my experience, almost half of adults feel compelled to eat everything on their plates, mainly because this was how they were brought up. Being a plate cleaner means you are responding to a visual cue rather than an internal hunger cue before you stop eating. Stop eating when you are full, and feel comfortable leaving food on your plate.

• **TV munchers.** Some people eat many of their meals in front of the TV or always like to nibble on a snack when watching their favourite programs. In this situation, you virtually have little knowledge of what, or how much, you eat. You have become distanced from the eating experience. Try eating your meals slowly at the dinner table. Eat with other people if possible, so that the table conversation helps slow down the rate at which you eat. If you do nibble while watching TV, make sure they are smart food choices such as fresh fruit, a whole-meal sandwich or roasted peanuts in the shell.

Food-Exercise Diary and Pedometers

Many health advisers suggest keeping a record of everything you eat and drink and all the exercise you do. This can be a very useful way of reminding you of your habits and whether you are on target for your goals. Sometimes it is really easy to forget the last time you went for a walk or to the gym. The diary can serve as a useful reminder.

Wearing a pedometer can also be very handy. This neat and inexpensive monitor can be worn on the belt and measures the number of steps taken each day. The aim for previously sedentary people is 7,000 steps daily, although this will need to increase to 10,000 to 12,000 steps for effective body fat loss and maintaining that loss.

Eating Disorders

Despite the impression that athletes are super healthy, the eating disorders anorexia nervosa and bulimia are common among athletes, especially females, who make up 90 per cent of those afflicted. It occurs mostly in women under pressure to be the perfect weight and shape in sports such as diving, gymnastics, distance running and synchronised swimming. Men who have to keep within a set weight or need to look very lean are also prone to eating disorders; for example, wrestlers, boxers, gymnasts and bodybuilders.

Eating habits can stray from normal long before the athlete gets stamped as having an eating disorder. Cutting back on food, occasional purging and other unhealthy habits to achieve weight loss may happen some time before an athlete becomes obsessed with the scales and skinfold callipers.

It isn't the purpose of this book to discuss how to prevent eating disorders, or how to solve them. All I can do is acknowledge their existence and point out some characteristics of eating disorders. If you suspect that you, or someone you know, has an eating disorder, I strongly recommend that you seek professional help or talk to an eating disorder support group.

Warning to Parents and Coaches

Parents and coaches can have a great impact on how athletes see themselves. Telling young athletes that they're fat or putting them on strict diets can lead to obsessive eating behaviour and eating disorders. Instead, suggest they see a sports dietitian who will give them the knowledge and guidance about nutrition to make changes that reduce body fat without reducing performance.

Anorexia Nervosa

Anorexia means 'without appetite'. This condition comes from not eating as a result of listening to outside sources that stress the importance of keeping a lean shape. It starts with dieting and becoming preoccupied with food, body weight and body shape. It is then followed by an enjoyment of dieting, periods of starvation and possibly a very high level of exercise to help weight loss. Sometimes the exercise is a form of punishment for eating too much.

Anorexic athletes can progress to being on a permanent diet and always thinking about food. They feel 'fat' while being thin. The body becomes emaciated and skinfold measurements are low. Often they become constipated and periods stop because of the lack of food. By this time they know the kilojoule content of every food in the supermarket. They may wear baggy or layers of clothing to hide their thinness and stay warm (they have too little insulating body fat to keep in the warmth).

Bulimia

People with bulimia are often on a strict diet, during which they sometimes eat lots and lots of food (binge eating), followed by purging through self-induced vomiting, laxatives or diuretics. People with bulimia usually eat very little in public, while tending to be closet eaters at home. They tend to visit the bathroom straight after eating. They may also engage in frequent vigorous exercise.

If vomiting is frequent, teeth repeatedly come into contact with stomach acids, causing erosion of the tooth enamel and eventual tooth decay. Often the family dentist is the first to suspect bulimia.

If you are preoccupied with food and constantly worrying about your weight, maybe it's time to call for help. To read more on this topic,

get the free fact sheet #14 ('Eating Disorders in Athletes') from www.sportsdietitians.com. Other resources include www.anred.com or the eating disorder group in your country, such as www.healthinsite.gov.au/topics/Eating_Disorders.

Female Triad Syndrome

With the pressure to maintain a very petite shape in many female athletes and dancers, they have to be mindful of everything they eat or drink. This can lead to food obsessions, strict dieting, inadequate intake of essential nutrients such as calcium and disordered eating. With very little food, the body reacts by ceasing menstrual loss (amenorrhea). The combination of disordered eating (anorexia or bulimia), amenorrhea and the loss of bone density is called the female triad syndrome.

Amenorrhea is not a normal and healthy response to training. The loss of periods results in a drop in estrogen and progesterone levels, infertility and often a loss of bone density. Estrogen and progesterone are hormones that protect against bone loss. Their levels drop to those of postmenopausal women during amenorrhea. If amenorrhea continues for many months, bone density may never return to normal.

A loss of bone density increases the risk of bone stress fractures and the early onset of osteoporosis (brittle bones) later in life. Exercise and an adequate consumption of calcium in the diet can help offset bone loss in this situation, but it is unlikely to stop it altogether.

The athlete with female triad syndrome should see a sports physician and be properly assessed. The long-term consequences of this syndrome are severe and can lead to irreversible bone damage and possibly death in extreme situations.

FINAL SCORE

- Your level of body fat can be assessed in a number of ways. Waist circumference, body mass index and skinfold measurements are the most common methods. Measuring your waist circumference is the easiest method for most athletes.
- Your metabolic rate will increase with extra training, an increase in muscle mass and possibly through dividing your meals into small, frequent snacks. Individual foods such as chilli, caffeine and green tea will have only a minor effect.

(continued)

- Diet books, diet plans, weight loss powders and pills, fat melters, exercise machines and any products promising quick weight loss are very unlikely to work in the long term.

- Sensible eating is the best route to long-term weight loss success. It means eating less saturated-fat-containing foods and more fruits, vegetables and whole-grain cereal foods.

- Choosing foods that have a low energy density (i.e., with the least amount of kilojoules or calories per 100 g) should be the basis of a fat loss eating plan.

- Be wary of overrestricting your food intake to meet a specified weight or shape. This could lead to disordered eating, inadequate nutrition and, for young women, female triad syndrome.

glossary

aerobic—Any activity that requires oxygen to be performed. In practical terms, this includes any activity that takes longer than 90 seconds. Aerobic activity will improve fitness and endurance, and will use both glucose (via glycogen) and fat as a fuel.

amino acids—The building blocks of protein. Just as house bricks can be constructed into a house, so amino acids can be constructed into proteins. Amino acids are classified as either dispensable (previously known as nonessential) or indispensable (previously known as essential). The body can make dispensable amino acids, whereas indispensable amino acids must be provided by the diet.

anabolic—Meaning 'to build up'. Growing through childhood and repairing a wound are examples of anabolism. The term *anabolic* is most commonly heard when referring to anabolic steroids, drugs that promote muscle buildup. Unfortunately, anabolic steroids have serious side effects.

anaerobic—Any activity that doesn't require oxygen to be performed. In practical terms, this includes any activity that takes less than 90 seconds, such as sprints and lifting weights. Some anaerobic activity is a part of most sports (e.g., a short sprint to catch a ball), but performing many sprints within a game will require aerobic fitness. Anaerobic activities use mainly glucose as a fuel.

ATP—Adenosine triphosphate. This molecule provides the energy for muscle contraction. ATP is manufactured from the metabolism of glucose.

carbohydrate—A combination of carbon, hydrogen and oxygen to form either starches (bread, rice, potato) or sugars (glucose, fructose, sucrose). Often abbreviated to 'carbs' or CHO (for carbon, hydrogen and oxygen).

Dietary Reference Intake (DRI)—A term used in the United States and Canada for the amount of each nutrient that will cover the health needs of virtually everyone. Because DRIs are set higher than the true needs of the body to give a margin of safety, they are not minimal requirements. The DRIs include the Recommended Dietary Allowances (RDAs) and Adequate Intakes (AI). The RDA is based on many years of research, while the AI is based on the best available data to date.

electrolyte drinks—Salts are electrolytes, and, in commercial terms, electrolyte drinks are those that contain sodium and potassium. Most will also contain carbohydrate in the form of sugars. Also known as sports drinks.

endurance—Usually, any continuous aerobic activity that takes longer than 60 minutes is a test of endurance fitness. The use of the term is subjective. Someone just starting a fitness program might find 30 minutes an endurance test.

ergogenic—A term commonly used to imply performance enhancing. It's from the Greek words *ergon* ('work') and *genesis* ('create'). Most nutritional ergogenic aids don't live up to their claims.

fat—Also known as *lipid*. A concentrated source of kilojoules that is found in many foods including oils (100 per cent fat), butter and margarine (80 per cent fat), cheese, biscuits, cakes, pastries, fried and deep-fried foods, many take-aways, sausages, salami, Devon, full-cream milk and yogurt.

glycogen—A chain of glucose molecules stored in the liver and muscles to be used as an efficient fuel for muscle contraction. Glycogen is manufactured from the carbohydrate foods in our diet. When glycogen stores are low, fatigue sets in as the body has to rely on the less efficient fat as a major fuel.

maximum heart rate—The heart rate, or pulse, that you achieve at your highest exercise intensity. It's about 220 beats per minute, minus your age in years as it will drop with age. It is commonly recommended that for fitness and good health you train at 60 to 80 per cent of your maximum heart rate, but this is a guide only and not a biological law.

If you are 30:

220 – 30 = 190

60 to 80% of 190 = 114 to 152

If you are 40:

220 – 40 = 180

60 to 80% of 180 = 108 to 144

mitochondria—Very small (20,000 laid end to end would be a millimetre) compartments in each cell of the body. They are the centre of energy production where ATP is transformed into energy. Larger numbers are found in muscle cells.

Nutrient Reference Values (NRV)—A term used in the United States, the United Kingdom, Canada, Australia and New Zealand. It includes the estimated average requirement or the adequate intake of essential nutrients. From this the Dietary Reference Intakes (which include the Recommended Daily Allowances in the United States and Canada), the Recommended Dietary Intakes (Australia and New Zealand) and the Reference Nutrient Intakes (UK) could be determined. The NRV also includes an upper intake limit above which the intake of a nutrient, usually as a supplement, could be detrimental to health.

osteopenia—Reduced bone mass. It can occur in female athletes who stop menstruating. Further bone loss can lead to early osteoporosis.

osteoporosis—A condition in which bone mass drops and bones become brittle and more likely to break as a result of minor injury.

placebo effect—The perceived positive effect of an inactive substance purely because the user believes in its value. The term *placebo* comes from the Latin word meaning 'I shall please'.

protein—An essential nutrient made from chains of amino acids. Protein is found in large amounts in meats, poultry, fish, cheese, yogurt, milk (but not butter) and eggs. About 30 per cent of the protein in our diet comes from bread, breakfast cereals, rice, pasta and legumes.

Recommended Dietary Allowances (RDA)—A term used in the United States and Canada for the amount of each nutrient that will cover the health needs of virtually everyone. Because they are set higher than the true needs of the body to give a margin of safety, they are not minimal requirements.

Recommended Dietary Intakes (RDI)—A term used in Australia and New Zealand for the amount of each nutrient that will cover the health needs of virtually everyone. Because they are set higher than the true needs of the body to give a margin of safety, they are not minimal requirements.

Reference Nutrient Intakes (RNI)—A term used in the United Kingdom for the amount of each nutrient that will cover the health needs of virtually everyone. Because they are set higher than the true needs of the body to give a margin of safety, they are not minimal requirements.

sodium—A mineral that is a part of salt (sodium chloride) and other food additives such as monosodium glutamate.

ultra-endurance events—Events for the committed athlete prepared to do many hours of training. The Ironman triathlon is a 3.8-kilometre (2.4-mile) swim, 180-kilometre (112-mile) bike ride, followed by a marathon (42 km or 26 miles).

conversion chart

Abbreviations

cal = calorie (in this book this is equivalent to a kilocalorie)
kJ = kilojoule
MJ = megajoule
fl oz = fluid ounce
mL = millilitre
L = litre
gal = gallon
oz = ounce
g = gram
lb = pound
kg = kilogram
ft = foot
yd = yard
c = centimeter
m = metre
km = kilometre
C = Celsius
F = Fahrenheit
hr = hour

Energy

1 cal (kilocalorie) = 4.18 kJ
1 kJ = 0.24 cal (kilocalorie)
1,000 kJ = 1 MJ (megajoule)

Volume

1 UK fl oz = 28.4 mL
1 US fl oz = 29.6 mL
1 mL = 0.034 fl oz
1 L = 0.22 UK gal
1 L = 0.26 US gal

Weight

1 oz = 28.35 g
1.5 oz = 42.5 g
12 oz = 340 g
1 g = 1,000 mg = 0.035 oz
1 lb = 0.45 kg
1 kg = 2.2 lb
55 kg = 121 lb
70 kg = 154 lb
90 kg = 198 lb
110 kg = 242 lb

Distance

1 inch = 2.5 cm
1 ft = 30.5 cm
1 yd = 91 cm
1 cm = 0.4 inch
1 m = 3 ft 3 inches
1 mile = 1.6 km
1 km = 0.62 mile

Temperature

Celsius = $0.555 \times (°\text{Fahrenheit} - 32)$
Fahrenheit = $(°\text{Celsius} \times 1.8) + 32$
20 °C = 68 °F
25 °C = 77 °F
30 °C = 86 °F
35 °C = 95 °F
100 °F = 37.8 °C
80 °F = 26.7 °C

Speed

1 km/hr = 0.62 miles/hr
1 mile/hr = 1.6 km/hr
60 km/hr = 37 miles/hr
100 km/hr = 62 miles/hr
40 miles/hr = 64 km/hr
100 miles/hr = 161 km/hr

nutrient food value chart

This chart provides a list of common foods with their protein, fat, carbohydrate and energy content. The alcohol content of common drinks is also included. Follow this list of foods as you record all that you eat and drink for a day, and gauge your protein, carbohydrate, fat and alcohol intake. I suggest you do this for three consecutive days and take a daily average. As new foods are constantly being released onto the market and other foods may be reformulated, you will also need to check labels for the nutrient profile. If you want to know the fat and kilojoule content of foods not listed, check the Web sites given at the end of the charts or go direct to the food company Web site as many now provide the nutrition information of all their products.

Note:

1. All numbers are in grams.
2. All measurements are metric (metric cups and spoons are available from supermarkets at little cost).
3. Spoon measurements are level (flat).
4. Numbers given are rounded numbers and in many cases can only be approximate values as the nutrition profile will vary depending on cooking method, processing method and brand name.

Food	Protein	Fat	Carbohydrate	Kilojoules	Calories
Fruit—fresh, canned, dried, juices					
Apple, canned, 1 cup	1	0	22	385	92
Apple, 1 med.	0	0	14	235	56
Apple juice, 200 mL	0	0	21	350	84
Apricot, canned, 1 cup	2	0	21	385	92
Apricot, dried, 1/2 cup	3	0	30	550	132
Apricot, 1 med.	0	0	4	65	16
Avocado, 1/2 med.	2	27	0	1,050	250
Banana, 1 med., peeled	2	0	22	400	96
Blackberry, canned, 1 cup	2	0	36	635	152
Blueberry, canned, 1 cup	2	0	41	720	172
Cherry, 10 (40 g)	0	0	5	85	20
Fig, dried, 2 pieces (30 g)	1	0	16	285	68
Fig, 1 med.	0	0	3	50	12
Fruit juice, av., 200 mL	0	0	20	335	80
Fruit salad, canned, 1 cup	1	0	24	420	100
Fruit salad, fresh, 1 cup	2	0	31	550	132

(continued)

171

(continued)

Food	Protein	Fat	Carbohydrate	Kilojoules	Calories
Fruit—fresh, canned, dried, juices					
Grapes, 1 cup	1	0	25	435	104
Grapefruit, 1/2	1	0	5	100	24
Grapefruit juice, 200 mL	1	0	12	215	52
Honeydew, no skin, 1 cup	1	0	11	200	48
Kiwi fruit, 1 med.	1	0	8	150	36
Lychees, canned, 1/2 cup	1	0	20	350	84
Mandarin, 1 med.	1	0	6	115	28
Mango, 1 med.	1	0	19	335	80
Mixed fruit, dried, 1 cup	3	1	98	1,730	413
Nectarine, 1 med.	1	0	6	115	28
Nectarine, canned, 1 cup	2	0	15	285	68
Orange, 1 med.	2	0	12	235	56
Orange juice, 200 mL	0	0	17	285	68
Paw paw, no skin, 1 cup	1	0	10	185	44
Peach, 1 med.	1	0	6	115	28
Peach, canned, 1 cup	2	0	19	350	84
Pear, 1 med.	0	0	18	300	72
Pear, canned, 1 half	0	0	6	100	24
Pineapple, canned, 1 ring	0	0	4	65	16
Pineapple, fresh, 1 sl.	1	0	9	165	40
Plum, 1 med.	0	0	6	100	24
Plum, canned, 1/2 cup	0	0	25	420	100
Prune, 10	2	0	35	620	148
Raspberry, canned, 1/2 cup	1	0	18	320	76
Rockmelon, 1 cup	1	0	8	150	36
Strawberry, 1 cup	2	0	4	100	24
Sultana, 1/4 cup	1	0	35	600	144
Tangerine, 1 med.	1	0	6	115	28
Watermelon, 1 cup	1	0	10	185	44
Breakfast cereals					
All-Bran, 1 cup	9	3	27	715	171
Branflakes, 1 cup	6	1	28	605	145
Breakfast bars—see snack foods					
Cornflakes, 1 cup	2	0	25	450	108
Fibre Plus, 1 cup	4	1	30	605	145
Fruity Bix, 10	3	1	29	575	137

Food	Protein	Fat	Carbohydrate	Kilojoules	Calories
Breakfast cereals					
Healthwise, 45 g	4	1	23	490	117
Just Right, 1 cup	4	1	36	705	169
Mini Wheats, 20 (40 g)	4	0	32	605	144
Muesli, Swiss style, 1 cup	15	12	65	1,790	428
Muesli, toasted 1 cup	9	15	50	1,555	371
Muesli, untoasted, 1 cup	7	7	45	1,135	271
Nutrigrain, 1 cup	6	0	22	470	112
Nut Feast, 45 g	4	4	26	655	156
Oat bran, 1 Tbsp	2	1	6	170	41
Porridge, 1 cup	4	3	20	515	123
Puffed Wheat, 1 cup	3	0	14	285	68
Rice Bubbles, 1 cup	1	0	18	320	76
Rolled oats, 1/2 cup	5	4	31	755	180
Shredded Wheat, 2	5	0	42	785	188
Special K, 1 cup	8	0	29	620	148
Sports Plus, 1 cup	4	1	32	640	153
Sustain, 1 cup	6	2	50	1,015	242
Weetabix, 2	5	1	27	570	134
Weetbix Multi-Grain, 2	5	3	32	730	175
Weetbix, Vita Brits, 2	4	1	20	440	105
Weeties, 1 cup	12	2	65	1,365	326
Wheat bran, unproc., 1 Tbsp	1	0	1	35	8
Legumes					
Baked beans, canned, 1 cup	10	1	25	625	149
Chickpeas, cooked, 1 cup	13	4	26	805	192
Kidney beans, canned, 1 cup	15	1	30	790	189
Lentils, boiled, 1 cup	14	1	19	590	141
3 bean mix, canned, 1 cup	14	1	30	775	185
Soybeans, canned, 1 cup	19	12	4	840	200
Vegetables					
Asparagus, 3 spears	0.5	0	2	42	10
Beans, green, 1/2 cup	0.5	0	2	42	10
Beetroot, 2 sl. av. (60 g)	1	0	5	100	24
Broccoli, 2 florets	1.5	0	1	42	10

(continued)

Food	Protein	Fat	Carbohydrate	Kilojoules	Calories
Vegetables					
Cabbage, 1/2 cup	0.5	0	1.5	35	8
Capsicum, 1/2 cup, chopped	1	0	1.5	42	10
Carrot, 1 cup	1	0	8	150	36
Cauliflower, 1/2 cup	2	0	2	70	16
Champignons, 1/2 cup	1	0	2	50	12
Cucumber, 4 sl., 30 g	0	0	1	17	4
Eggplant, 2 sl., 60 g	0.5	0	1.5	35	8
French fries, 100 g	4	15	20	965	231
Lettuce, 1 cup, shredded	0.5	0	0.5	17	4
Mushrooms, 1/2 cup	1.5	0	1	42	10
Mushrooms, canned, butter sauce	1.5	1	5	145	35
Peas, green, cooked, 1 cup	9	1	9	340	81
Parsnip, cooked, 1/2 cup	1	0	7	135	32
Potato, boiled, 1 med. (120 g)	3	0	16	320	76
Potato, baked, 1 med.	3	8	16	620	148
Potato, mashed, 1 cup	6	1	30	640	153
Potato chips, 100 g	4	7	20	665	159
Potato chips, 10 oven fries	3	4	24	605	144
Potato wedges, 100 g	4	9	20	740	177
Pumpkin, boiled, 1 cup	6	2	18	475	114
Pumpkin, baked, 100 g	7	7	22	750	179
Sweet potato, cooked, 1 cup	4	0	40	735	176
Sweetcorn, kernels, 1 cup	5	2	30	660	158
Tomato, 1 med. (100 g)	1	0	2	50	12
Zucchini, 100 g	1	0	2	50	12
Rice and pasta					
Continental Rice meal, av., 1 cup	7	5	52	1,175	281
Pasta, boiled, 1 cup	8	1	50	1,010	241
Rice, steamed, 1 cup	5	1	50	960	229
Spaghetti, canned, 1 cup	5	1	30	625	149
Tortellini, cheese and spinach, 1 cup	16	8	58	1,540	368
Rice cakes, 1	1	0	10	185	44

Food	Protein	Fat	Carbohydrate	Kilojoules	Calories
Rice and pasta sauces					
Chicken Tonight, 1/2 cup, av.	2	5	10	390	93
Coconut milk, lite, 50 mL	0	7	2	295	71
Dolmio, chunky, 1/2 cup, av.	2	0	14	270	64
Dolmio, heat and serve, 1/2 cup, av.	2	2	10	275	66
Leggo's, stir through, av. serve	2	8	8	400	96
Breads, biscuits and cakes					
Breads					
Bread, 1 sl. (30 g)	3	1	15	340	81
Bread roll, 1 med. (60 g)	6	1	27	590	141
Crumpet, 1	3	0	20	385	92
Fruit bun, 1 med. (80 g)	7	3	40	900	215
Fruit bread, 1 sl. (30 g)	2	1	15	320	77
Garlic bread, 2 sl.	6	10	32	1,015	242
Lebanese bread, 1 circle	10	3	57	1,235	295
Muffin, English style, 1 (80 g)	7	1	28	625	149
Scone, av. (50 g)	4	5	25	675	161
Cakes					
Black forest cake, 100 g	4	19	40	1,450	347
Cheesecake, lg. sl. (120 g)	5	23	42	1,655	395
Fruit cake, 1 sl. (50 g)	2	5	28	690	165
Lamington, 1 (75 g)	4	9	36	860	205
Mudcake, 100 g	3	16	38	1,290	308
Rock cake, av. (50 g)	3	8	29	835	200
Swiss roll, 1 sl. (30 g)	1	2	19	410	98
Vanilla slice, 130 g	4	15	35	1,220	291
Biscuits, crackers					
Biscuit, ginger, 1	0	1	7	155	37
Biscuit, plain, sweet, 1	1	2	7	210	50
Crispbread, 2 av.	1	0	8	150	36
Digestive biscuit, 20 g	1	4	14	365	87
Pretzels, 20 sticks	1	1	8	190	45
Rice crackers, 10	1	0	14	250	60
Ryvita, 2	2	0	13	250	60
Water crackers, 4 av.	2	2	12	475	114

(continued)

(continued)

Food	Protein	Fat	Carbohydrate	Kilojoules	Calories
Breads, biscuits and cakes					
Pastry, pies					
Apple pie, 150 g	4	15	40	1,300	311
Croissant, 65 g	7	15	23	1,065	255
Danish pastry, 1	8	16	36	1,340	320
Donut, 50 g	3	10	20	760	182
Flour, 1 cup, av.	16	2	85	1,765	422
Dairy foods, soy milk, tofu					
Brie, Camembert, 30 g	6	8	0	400	96
Cheese, hard, av., 30 g	7	9	0	455	109
Cottage cheese, 30 g	4	2	0	140	34
Cream cheese, 30 g	3	10	1	475	114
Feta, 30 g	5	7	0	345	83
Ice cream, 1 scoop	2	5	10	390	93
Milk, skim/nonfat, 200 mL	8	0	12	335	80
Milk, reduced fat, 200 mL	8	4	12	485	116
Milk, whole, 200 mL	7	8	9	570	136
Milk, evaporated, 200 mL	16	16	23	1,255	300
Milk, evaporated skim, 200 mL	16	1	23	690	165
Milk, flavoured, 300 mL, av.	12	6	25	845	202
Milk powder, whole, 3 Tbsp	8	8	11	620	148
Milk powder, skim, 3 Tbsp	11	0	15	435	104
Parmesan, 30 g	11	9	0	525	125
Processed cheese, av., 30 g	6	8	0	400	96
Ricotta, quark, 30 g	3	3	1	180	43
Yogurt, skim, plain, 200 mL	14	0	12	435	104
Yogurt, skim, flavoured, 200 mL	10	0	26	605	144
Yogurt, reg., plain, 200 mL	12	9	9	690	165
Yogurt, reg., flavoured, 200 mL	9	4	25	720	172
Soy products					
So Good, 200 mL	7	7	9	575	137
So Good Lite, 200 mL	7	1	12	355	85
So Good, flavoured, 200 mL	7	6	14	580	138
Tofu, firm 100 g	5	2	6	260	62
Tofu, Thai style, 100 g	18	9	5	1,725	173

Food	Protein	Fat	Carbohydrate	Kilojoules	Calories
Drinks					
Cordial (1:4 dilute), 200 mL	0	0	15	250	60
Drinking chocolate powder, 25 g	1	1.5	20	410	98
Dry ginger ale, 200 mL	0	0	17	285	68
Energy drinks, 250 mL	0	0	27	450	108
Flavoured milks, 300 mL	12	6	25	845	202
Fruit juice, av., 250 mL	0	0	30	500	120
Fruit juice drinks, 250 mL	0	0	30	500	120
Gatorade, 500 mL	0	0	30	500	120
Horlicks powder, 25 g	2.5	1	20	415	99
Lucozade Sport, 500 mL	0	0	32	530	128
Milo, Aktavite, Ovaltine, av., 1 Tbsp, 10 g	1	1	6	140	33
Mineral water, flavoured, 375 mL	0	0	42	705	168
Powerade, 500 mL	0	0	40	670	160
Soft drink, diet, 375 mL	0	0	0	0	0
Sports water, 250 mL	0	0	6	100	24
Sports water, low joule, 250 mL	0	0	0	0	0
Soda water, 200 mL	0	0	0	0	0
Soft drink, av., 375 mL	0	0	40	670	160
Sports drink, av., 500 mL	0	0	30	500	120
Staminade, 250 mL	0	0	13	220	52
Sustagen Sport, 1 Tbsp, 10 g	2	0	7	150	36
Sustagen Sport, 250 mL	18	0	49	1,120	268
Tonic water, 200 mL	0	0	17	285	68
Velvet chocolate flakes, 25 g	2	6	14	495	118
Water, plain mineral	0	0	0	0	0
Snack foods					
Solid snacks					
Apricots, 5, dried	1	0	15	270	64
Breakfast bar, av.	2	3	28	615	147
Cereal bar, av.	2	0.5	27	500	120
Fresh fruit, av.	1	0	15	270	64
Fruesli Bar, 45 g, av.	1.5	1.5	28	550	131
Fruit bars, 50 g, av.	1	0	30	520	124

(continued)

(continued)

Food	Protein	Fat	Carbohydrate	Kilojoules	Calories
Solid snacks					
Fruit bun, 1 med.	7	3	40	900	215
Fruity bix bar (Sanitarium)	2	2.5	18	425	102
Jelly beans, 10	0	0	30	500	120
Marathon bar, 55 g, av.	11	7	54	1,350	323
Potato crisps, 50 g	3	16	24	1,055	252
Power bar	10	2	42	945	226
Raisin bread, 1 sl.	2	.1	15	320	77
Rice crackers, 1	1	0	10	185	44
Sultanas, 1/4 cup	1	0	35	605	144
Uncle Tobys oven baked fruit bar, av.	1	1	29	540	129
Uncle Tobys muesli bar, av.	2	3	22	515	123
Uncle Tobys Twist bar, av.	2	1	30	575	137
Desserts and yogurts					
Frûche, 1 carton, 130 g	10	4	19	635	152
Frûche Lite, 1 carton, 130 g	8	1	18	440	105
Fromais, reg., 175 g	6	10	33	1,030	246
Fromais, light, 175 g	8	2	26	645	154
Ice cream, 2 scoops	4	10	20	780	186
Ski Double Up, 200 g	8	1.5	36	790	189
Yogurt, reg., 200 g	10	6	32	930	222
Yogurt, low fat, 200 g	10	0	36	770	184
Yogurt, diet, 200 g	10	0	14	400	96
Yo-Split, 200 g	9	3	41	950	227
Yoplait, reg., 200 g	9	2	16	495	118
Yoplait, light, 200 g	10	0	16	435	104
Yogurt, nonfat, flavoured, 200 mL	10	0	26	605	144
Jam, marmalade, jelly					
Glucodin, 1 Tbsp	0	0	16	270	64
Honey, 1 Tbsp	0	0	22	370	88
Jelly, reg., 1/2 cup	2	0	19	350	84
Jelly, low joule, 1/2 cup	2	0	0	33	8
Marmalade, jam, 1 Tbsp	0	0	14	235	56
Mayonnaise, 1 Tbsp	0	6	4	295	70
Popcorn, 1 cup	1	2	4	115	28
Sugar, glucose, 1 tsp	0	0	4	65	16
Vegemite, 1 tsp	1	0	0	17	4

Food	Protein	Fat	Carbohydrate	Kilojoules	Calories
Fat and oils					
Butter, 1 Tbsp	0	16	0	600	144
Copha, 1 Tbsp	0	20	0	755	180
Margarine, reg., 1 Tbsp	0	16	0	600	144
Margarine, reduced fat, 1 Tbsp	0	8	0	300	72
Oils, 1 Tbsp	0	20	0	755	180
Nuts and seeds					
Almonds, 25 g	4	13	1	575	137
Brazil nuts, walnuts, 25 g	3	17	0	690	165
Cashews, 25 g	4	13	4	625	149
Peanut butter, 1 Tbsp (30 g)	7	15	3	735	175
Peanuts, 25 g	6	12	3	605	144
Sesame seeds, 30 g	6	15	0	665	159
Sunflower seeds, 30 g	7	14	0	645	154
Tahini, 30 g	6	18	0	780	186
Eggs, meat, chicken and seafood					
Black pudding, 100 g	10	22	17	1,255	300
Chicken, leg, lean, 100 g	27	10	0	830	198
Chicken, breast, lean, 100 g	28	5	0	655	157
Crab, 100 g	12	1	0	240	57
Egg, 1 whole	7	6	0	345	82
Egg white, from 1 egg, 40 g	4	0	0	67	16
Egg yolk, from 1 egg, 20 g	3	6	0	276	66
Fish, av., cooked, 100 g	22	5	0	555	133
Fish, canned, 100 g, brine	22	5	0	555	133
Fish, canned, 100 g, oil	22	15	0	935	223
Ham, canned/cured, 30 g	5	2	0	160	38
Lobster, prawn, 100 g	22	1	0	405	97
Luncheon meats, av., 30 g	4	10	0	445	106
Meat, lean, av., cooked, 100 g	27	8	0	755	180
Mussels, 12 boiled	20	2	0	410	98
Oysters, 6 raw	6	1	0	140	33
Paté, 1 Tbsp (20 g)	4	5	0	255	61
Pork pie, 100 g	11	26	24	1,520	365
Sausage, 100 g	15	20	5	1,090	260
Scallops, 6 steamed	13	1	0	255	61

(continued)

(continued)

Food	Protein	Fat	Carbohydrate	Kilojoules	Calories
Eggs, meat, chicken and seafood					
Scotch egg, 100 g	12	16	13	1,005	240
Tuna, canned, salsa, 100 g	19	5	3	555	133
Tuna, canned, Thai, 100 g	18	11	5	800	191
Sauces, gravy					
Barbeque sauce, 1 Tbsp	0	0	9	150	36
Chilli sauce, 1 Tbsp	0	0	4	65	16
Gravy, commercial, 1 Tbsp	1	2	2	125	30
Soy sauce, 1 Tbsp	1	0	0.5	25	6
Tomato sauce, 1 Tbsp	0	0	5	85	20
Tartare sauce, 30 mL	0	8	4	370	88
Worcestershire sauce, 1 Tbsp	0	0	4	65	16
Take-aways					
Subway					
Chicken Fillet Classic Salad, 6 in.	16	14	11	960	229
Chicken Satay, 6 in.	18	9	50	1,500	560
Italian BMT, 6 in.	22	25	44	2,040	485
Southwest Turkey Bacon Melt, 6 in.	18	18	48	1,770	422
Subway Club, 6 in.	18	6	44	1,240	295
Tuna Salad, 6 in.	13	9	16	820	195
Turkey Breast, 6 in.	15	6	43	1,210	290
Veggie Delite, 6 in.	9	4	42	990	235
Hungry Jacks					
Chicken nuggets, 7 pack	21	28	24	1,810	432
Double bacon cheeseburger	41	40	34	2,765	660
Fries, reg.	4	18	43	1,465	350
Fries, lg.	6	25	59	2,030	485
Shake, reg.	6.5	8	53	1,300	310
Whopper	24	34	52	2,555	610
Red Rooster					
Chicken and chips	29	47	83	3,645	871
Chicken roll	22	13	59	1,845	441
Hawaiian pack	29	51	91	3,930	939
Skin-free, 200 g	50	13	4	1,395	333

Food	Protein	Fat	Carbohydrate	Kilojoules	Calories
Take-aways					
Chicken Treat					
Chicken dinner	51	26	65	2,920	698
Chicken fillet burger	24	17	48	1,245	297
Wedges, large, 440 g	16	46	113	3,895	930
Taco Bell					
Beef Enchirito	12	9	35	1,130	270
Chalupa supreme beef	14	24	31	1,630	390
Chicken burrito supreme	19	8	50	1,465	350
Chilli cheese burrito	16	18	40	1,630	390
Double decker taco supreme	15	18	41	1,590	380
Gordita supreme steak	16	19	28	1,215	290
Nachos	5	19	33	1,340	320
Soft taco, beef	10	10	21	880	210
McDonald's					
Bacon & Egg McMuffin	17	15	25	1,270	303
Big Mac	25	30	46	2,340	560
Cheeseburger	15	12	35	1,295	310
Chicken Foldover	29	9	48	1,630	389
Filet-o-fish	14	18	42	1,670	400
French fries, sm.	2	11	30	960	230
French fries, med.	4	16	47	1,465	350
French fries, lg.	6	25	70	2,175	520
Garden Mixed Salad	6	4	2	285	68
Junior burger	13	9	32	1,095	261
McFlurry, av.	10	14	60	1,700	406
McNuggets, 6	15	15	15	1,045	250
Milkshake, med.	13	10	58	1,565	374
Quarter pounder with cheese	34	28	37	2,245	536
Roast Chicken Salad	16	7	20	865	207
Sausage McMuffin	14	21	31	1,550	370
Vege Burger	16	10	55	1,565	374
KFC					
Breast	20	15	7	1,045	250
Caesar Salad without dressing	29	6	6	920	220
Chicken Fillet Burger	30	17	28	1,225	295

(continued)

(continued)

Food	Protein	Fat	Carbohydrate	Kilojoules	Calories
KFC					
Chicken nuggets, with sauce, 6	18	17	20	1,255	300
Drumstick	13	8	4	585	140
Fries/chips, lg.	10	40	65	2,710	645
Hot Wings, 6	24	29	23	1,885	450
Mashed potato and gravy	4	2	12	335	80
Thigh	18	22	5	1,210	290
Wing, whole, plain	11	9	5	630	150
Pizza Hut					
Pan Pizza					
Cheese, 1 sl.	14	10	29	1,095	262
Hawaiian, 1 sl.	15	11	36	1,270	303
Super Supreme, 1 sl.	18	15	35	1,450	347
Supreme, 1 sl.	19	16	32	1,455	348
Thin 'n Crispy Pizza					
Cheese, 1 sl.	13	9	22	925	221
Hawaiian, 1 sl.	14	10	26	1,045	250
Super Supreme, 1 sl.	17	14	26	1,415	338
Supreme, 1 sl.	17	13	27	1,225	293
Other take-aways					
Cheesecake, 1 piece	6	22	30	1,430	342
Fish, battered, 1 piece	21	23	20	1,555	371
French fries, reg.	5	23	52	1,820	435
Hot potato chips	4	13	25	975	233
Meat pie	15	26	34	1,800	430
Meat pie, party size	3	7	8	450	107
Sausage roll, lg.	10	23	32	1,570	375
Sausage roll, party size	4	8	8	500	120
Wedges, reg.	4	20	50	1,660	396
Confectionery					
Boiled lollies, 1 av.	0	0	5	85	20
Chocolate, dark, 100 g	5	29	63	2,230	533
Chocolate, milk, 100 g	8	28	57	2,145	512
Cadbury Lite, 100 g	5	28	7	1,255	300
Chocolate, milk, with nuts, 100 g	11	30	53	2,200	526
Caramello, 100 g	6	22	62	1,965	470

Food	Protein	Fat	Carbohydrate	Kilojoules	Calories
Confectionery					
Jelly beans, 1	0	0	3	50	12
Jelly snakes, 1	0	0	4	67	16
Mars bar, 60 g	2	11	42	1,150	275
Mars bar lite, 45 g	2	5	29	705	169
Snickers bar, 60 g	6	13	36	1,195	285
Turkish Delight, 55 g	1	5	40	875	209

For More Information on the Nutrition Content of Foods

Web Sites

Australia and New Zealand

www.calorieking.com.au/foods/?partner=hwf

United States

www.calorie-count.com/

www.nal.usda.gov/fnic/foodcomp/search/ (The United States Department of Agriculture National Nutrient Database)

Books

Australia and New Zealand

Borushek, A. 2006. *Calorie, fat & carbohydrate counter.* Nedlands: Family Health Publications.

Food Standards Australia and New Zealand. 1997. *Nutritional values of Australian foods.* Canberra: Australian Government Publishing Service.

United Kingdom

Food Standards Agency. 2002. *McCance and Widdowson's the composition of foods.* 6th summary ed. Cambridge: Royal Society of Chemistry.

Sims, J. and T. Walton. 2005. *The calorie, carb & fat bible.* Oxford: Penhaligon Page.

United States

Borushek, A. 2005. *The doctor's pocket calorie, fat & carb counter.* Costa Mesa, CA: Family Health Publications.

Pennington, J.A.T., and J.S. Douglass. 2005. *Bowes and Church's food values of portions commonly used.* 18th ed. Baltimore: Lippincott, Williams and Wilkins.

bibliography

chapter one

Australian Bureau of Statistics. 1998. *National nutrition survey: Nutrient intakes and physical measurements*. Canberra: Commonwealth of Australia.

Kirkendall, D.T. 1993. Effects of nutrition on performance in soccer. *Medicine & Science in Sports & Exercise* 25 (12): 1370-1374.

McNab, Tom. 1980. The complete book of track and field. New York: Exeter Books p. 73.

Mann, J., and A.S. Truswell. 2002. *Essentials of human nutrition*. Oxford: Oxford University Press.

Manore, M., and J. Thompson. 2000. *Sport nutrition for health and performance*. Champaign, IL: Human Kinetics.

Sherwood, L. 2001. *Human physiology*. 4th ed. Pacific Grove, CA: Brooks/Cole.

Valtin, H. 2002. 'Drink at least eight glasses of water a day'. Really? Is there scientific evidence for '8 × 8'? *American Journal of Physiology* 283:R993-R1004.

Whitney, E.R., and S.R. Rolfes. 2005. *Understanding nutrition*. 10th ed. Belmont, CA: Wadsworth.

chapter two

Antonio, J., and J.R. Stout. 2002. *Supplements for strength-power athletes*. Champaign, IL: Human Kinetics.

Brill, J.B., and M.W. Keane. 1994. Supplementation patterns of competitive male and female bodybuilders. *International Journal of Sport Nutrition* 4:398-412.

Davis, J.M. 1995. Carbohydrates, branched-chain amino acids, and endurance: The central fatigue hypothesis. *International Journal of Sport Nutrition* 5:S29-S38.

Evans, W.J. 2001. Protein nutrition and resistance exercise. *Canadian Journal of Applied Physiology* 26 (Suppl): S141-S152.

Fogelholm, G.M., H.K. Näveri, K.T.K. Kiilavuori and M.H.A. Härkönen. 1993. Low-dose amino acid supplementation: No effects on serum human growth hormone and insulin in male weightlifters. *International Journal of Sport Nutrition* 3:290-297.

Fricker, P.A., S.K. Beasley and I.W. Copeland. 1988. Physiological growth hormone responses of throwers to amino acids, eating and exercise. *Australian Journal of Science and Medicine in Sport* (March):21-23.

Lambert, M.I., J.A. Hefer, R.P. Millar and P.W. Macfarlane. 1993. Failure of commercial oral amino acid supplements to increase serum growth hormone concentrations in male bodybuilders. *International Journal of Sport Nutrition* 3:298-305.

Lemon, P.W.R. 1998. Effects of exercise on dietary protein requirements. *International Journal of Sport Nutrition* 8: 426-447.

Manninen, A.H. 2004. Protein hydrolysates in sports and exercise: A brief review. *Journal of Sports Science and Medicine* 3:60-63.

Mero, A. 1999. Leucine supplementation and intensive training. *Sports Medicine* 27:347-358.

Millward, D.J. 1999. Optimal intakes of protein in the human diet. *Proceedings of the Nutrition Society* 58: 403-413.

Mittleman, K.D., M.R. Ricci and S.P. Bailey. 1998. Branched-chain amino acids prolong exercise during heat stress in men and women. *Medicine & Science in Sports & Exercise* 30:83-91.

Saunders, M.J., M.D. Kane and M.K. Todd. 2004. Effects of a carbohydrate-protein beverage on cycling endurance and muscle damage. *Medicine & Science in Sports & Exercise* 36:1233-1238.

Silk, D.B.A. 1980. Use of a peptide rather than free amino acid nitrogen source in chemically defined 'elemental' diets. *Journal of Parenteral and Enteral Nutrition* 4 (6): 548-553.

Tarnopolsky, M. 2000. Protein and amino acid needs for training and bulking up. In *Clinical sports nutrition*. L. Burke and V. Deakin, eds. Sydney: McGraw-Hill, p. 112.

Tipton, K.D., and R.R. Wolfe. 2001. Exercise, protein metabolism, and muscle growth. *International Journal of Sport Nutrition and Exercise Metabolism* 11:109-132.

Walberg-Rankin, J. 1995. A review of nutritional practices and needs of bodybuilders. *Journal of Strength and Conditioning Research* 9 (2):116-124.

chapter three

Augustin, L.S., S. Franceschi, D.J.A. Jenkins, C.W.C. Kendall and C. la Vecchia. 2002. Glycemic index in chronic disease: A review. *European Journal of Clinical Nutrition* 56:1049-1071.

Bergström, J., and E. Hultman. 1967. Muscle glycogen synthesis after exercise: An enhancing factor localised to the muscle cells in man. *Nature* 210:309-310.

Brand-Miller, J., K. Foster-Powell and S. Colagiuri. 2002. *The new glucose revolution*. London: Hodder.

Burke, L.M., G.R. Collier and M. Hargreaves. 1998. Glycemic index—A new tool in sports nutrition? *International Journal of Sport Nutrition* 8:401-415.

Carbohydrate in human nutrition. 1997. Interim Report of a Joint FAO/WHO Expert Consultation. Food & Agriculture Organization of the United Nations.

DeMarco, H.M., K.P. Sucher, C.J Cisar and G.E. Butterfield. 1999. Pre-exercise carbohydrate meals: Application of the glycemic index. *Medicine & Science in Sports & Exercise* 31:164-170.

Egger, G., and B. Swinburn. 1996. *Fat loss leaders handbook.* London: Allen and Unwin.

Flatt, J.-P. 1995. Use and storage of carbohydrate and fat. *American Journal of Clinical Nutrition* 61 (Suppl): 952S-959S.

Foster-Powell, K.S., H.A. Holt and J.C. Brand-Miller. 2002. International table of glycemic index and glycemic load values: 2002. *American Journal of Clinical Nutrition* 76: 5-56.

Hawley, J.A., and L.M. Burke. 1997. Effect of meal frequency and timing on physical performance. *British Journal of Nutrition* 77 (Suppl):S91-S103.

Kolkhorst, F.W., J.N. MacTaggart and M.R. Hansen. 1998. Effect of a sports food bar on fat utilisation and exercise duration. *Canadian Journal of Applied Physiology* 23: 271-278.

McWhirter, N., ed. 1980. *Guinness Book of Records.* 27th ed. Middlesex: Guinness Superlatives Ltd.

Sherwood, S. 2001. *Human physiology.* 4th ed. Pacific Grove, CA: Brooks/Cole.

chapter four

American College of Sports Medicine. 2000. Nutrition and athletic performance. *Medicine & Science in Sports & Exercise.* 32:2130-2145.

Beard, J. 2002. Iron status and exercise. *American Journal of Clinical Nutrition* 72 (Suppl):594S-597S.

Burke, L., and V. Deakin, eds. 2000. *Clinical sports nutrition.* 2nd ed. New York: McGraw-Hill, pp. 312-334.

Burke, L.M., E. Coyle and R. Maughan. 2004. *Nutrition for athletes.* Lausanne, Switzerland: International Olympic Committee Medical Commission Working Group on Sports Nutrition.

Clarkson, P. 1995. Antioxidants and physical performance. *Critical Reviews in Food Science and Nutrition* 35 (1 and 2):131-141.

Cobiac, L., and K. Baghurst. 1993. Iron status and dietary iron intakes of Australians. *Food Australia* (Suppl) April.

Executive summary of nutrient reference values for Australia and New Zealand. 2005. Canberra: Commonwealth of Australia and New Zealand Government.

Fogelholm, M. 1994. Vitamins, minerals and supplementation in soccer. *Journal of Sports Sciences* 12:S23-S27.

Hallberg, L., and L. Hulthén. 2000. Prediction of dietary iron absorption: An algorithm for calculating absorption and bioavailability of dietary iron. *American Journal of Clinical Nutrition* 71:1147-1160.

Haymes, E.M. 1991. Vitamin and mineral supplementation to athletes. *International Journal of Sport Nutrition* 1:146-169.

Nielsen, P., and D. Nachtigall. 1998. Iron supplementation in athletes. *Sports Medicine* 26:207-216.

Peake, J.M. 2003. Vitamin C: Effects of exercise and requirements with training. *International Journal of Sport Nutrition and Exercise Metabolism* 13:125-151.

Report of the Panel on Dietary Reference Values of the Committee on Medical Aspects of Food Policy. 1991. London: Her Majesty's Stationery Office.

Sports Dietitians Australia. 2000. Fact sheet #10: Bone health. Melbourne: Sports Dietitians Australia.

Sports Dietitians Australia. 2002. Fact sheet #16: Iron depletion in athletes. Melbourne: Sports Dietitians Australia.

Telford, R.D. 1992. The effect of 7 to 8 months of vitamin/mineral supplementation on athletic performance. *International Journal of Sport Nutrition* 2:135-153.

Tiidus, P.M. and M.E. Houston. 1995. Vitamin E status and response to exercise training. *Sports Medicine* 20 (1): 12-23.

van der Beek, E.J. 1991. Vitamin supplementation and physical exercise performance. *Journal of Sports Sciences* 9:77-89.

Wahlqvist, M.L., ed. 2002. *Food and nutrition.* London: Allen and Unwin.

chapter five

2005 Fact sheets. 2005. *Australian Institute of Sport.* www.ais.org.au/nutrition/HotTopics.asp.

Armstrong, L.E., D.L. Costill and W.J. Fink. 1985. Influence of diuretic-induced dehydration on competitive running performance. *Medicine & Science in Sports & Exercise* 14:456-461.

Australian Institute of Health and Welfare. 2004. *Australia's health 2004.* Canberra: Australian Institute of Health and Welfare.

Bar-Or, O. 1994. Children's responses to exercise in hot climates: Implications for performance and health. *Sports Science Exchange* 77 (2).

Barr, S.I., and D.L. Costill. 1989. Water: Can the endurance athlete get too much of a good thing? *Journal of the American Dietetic Association* 89:1629-1632, 1635.

Bergeron, M.F. 1996. Heat cramps during tennis: A case report. *International Journal of Sport Nutrition* 6:62-68.

Brouns, F., J. Senden, E.J. Beckers and W.H.M. Saris. 1995. Osmolarity does not effect the gastric emptying rate of oral rehydration solutions. *Journal of Parenteral and Enteral Nutrition* 19 (5):403-406.

Burke, L.M. 1996. Rehydration strategies before and after exercise. *Australian Journal of Nutrition and Dietetics* 53 (4 Suppl):S22-S26.

Cox, G.R., E.M. Broad, M.D. Riley and L.M. Burke. 2002. Body mass changes and voluntary fluid intakes of elite level water polo players and swimmers. *Journal of Science and Medicine in Sport* 5 (3):183-193.

Davis, M.J., D.A. Jackson, M.S. Broadwell, J.L. Queary and C.L. Lambert. 1997. Carbohydrate drinks delay fatigue during intermittent, high-intensity cycling in active men and women. *International Journal of Sport Nutrition* 7:261-273.

Epstein, Y., and L.E. Armstrong. 1999. Fluid-electrolyte balance during labor and exercise: Concepts and misconceptions. *International Journal of Sport Nutrition* 9: 1-12.

Fixx J. 1978. *Jim Fixx's Second Book of Running*. New York: Random House.

Gardner, J.W. 2002. Death by water intoxication. *Military Medicine* 167 (5):432-434.

Gisolfi, C.V. 1995. Effect of sodium concentration in a carbohydrate-electrolyte solution on intestinal absorption. *Medicine & Science in Sports & Exercise* 27: 1414-1420.

Gore, C.J., P.C. Bourdon, S.M. Woolford and D.G. Pederson. 1993. Involuntary dehydration during cricket. *International Journal of Sports Medicine* 14:387-395.

Gutierrez, G. 1995. Solar injury and heat illness: Treatment and prevention in children. *Physician and Sportsmedicine* 23 (7):43-48.

Hargreaves, M. 1996. Physiological benefits of fluid and energy replacement during exercise. *Australian Journal of Nutrition and Dietetics* 53 (4 Suppl):S3-S7.

Hew-Butler T., C. Almond, J.C.Ayus, J. Dugas, W. Meeuwisse, T. Noakes, S. Reid, A. Siegal, D. Speedy, K. Stuempfle, J. Verbalis, L. Weschler. 2005. Consensus Statement of the 1st International Exercise-Associated Hyponatremia Consensus Development Conference, Cape Town, South Africa 2005. *Clinical Journal of Sports Medicine* 15: 208-213.

Institute of Medicine, Food and Nutrition Board. 2004. Press Release. www4.nationalacademies.org/news.nsf/ isbn/0309091691?opendocument.

Luetkemeier, M.J., M.G. Coles and E.W. Askew. 1997. Dietary sodium and plasma volume levels with exercise. *Sports Medicine* 23:279-286.

Lyle, D.M., P.R. Lewis, D.A.B. Richards, R. Richards, A.E. Bauman, J.R. Sutton and I.D. Cameron. 1994. Heat exhaustion in the Sun-Herald City to Surf fun run. *Medical Journal of Australia* 161:361-365.

Maughan, R.J. 1998. The sports drink as a functional food: Formulations for successful performance. *Proceedings of the Nutrition Society* 57:1-10.

Maughan, R.J., and J.B. Leiper. 1995. Sodium intake and post-exercise rehydration in man. *European Journal of Applied Physiology and Occupational Physiology* 71 (4): 311-319.

Maughan, R.J., and N.J. Rehrer. 1993. Gastric emptying during exercise. *Gatorade Sports Science Institute* 6 (5).

Millward A, L. Shaw, E. Harrington, A.J. Smith. 1997. Continuous monitoring of salivary flow rate and pH at the surface of the dentition following consumption of acidic beverages. *Caries Research* 31: 44-49.

Milosevic A. 1997. Sports drinks hazard to teeth. *British Journal of Sports Medicine* 31: 28-30 (see also responses: Brouns, F., and L. Muntjewerf. Sports drinks and teeth. *British Journal of Sports Medicine* 31:258 and Murray, R. 1997. Sports drinks and teeth. *British Journal of Sports Medicine* 31:352).

Morton, D.P., and R. Callister. 2000. Characteristics and etiology of exercise-related transient abdominal pain. *Medicine & Science in Sports & Exercise* 32:432-438.

Morton, D.P., and R. Callister. 2002. Factors influencing exercise-related transient abdominal pain. *Medicine & Science in Sports & Exercise* 34:745-749.

Moss SJ. 1998. Dental erosion. *International Dental Journal* 48: 529-539.

Murray, R. 1996. Guidelines for fluid replacement during exercise. *Australian Journal of Nutrition and Dietetics* 53 (4 Suppl):S17-S21.

National Health and Medical Research Council. 2003. Dietary guidelines for Australian adults. A guide to healthy eating.

Passe, D.H., M. Horn and R. Murray. 1997. The effects of beverage carbonation on sensory responses and voluntary fluid intake following exercise. *International Journal of Sport Nutrition* 7:286-297.

Ploutz-Snyder, L., J. Foley, R. Ploutz-Snyder, J. Kanaley, K. Sagendorf and R. Meyer. 1999. Gastric gas and fluid emptying assessed by magnetic resonance imaging. *European Journal of Applied Physiology and Occupational Physiology* 79:212-220.

Plunkett, B.T., and W.G. Hopkins. 1999. Investigation of the side pain "stitch"induced by running after fluid ingestion. *Medicine & Science in Sports & Exercise* 31: 1169-1175.

Rehrer, N.J. 1996. Factors influencing fluid bioavailability. *Australian Journal of Nutrition and Dietetics* 53 (4 Suppl): S8-S12.

Rehrer, N.J., and L.M. Burke. 1996. Sweat losses during various sports. *Australian Journal of Nutrition and Dietetics* 53 (4 Suppl):S13-S16.

Saunders, M.J., M.D. Kane and M.K. Todd. 2004. Effects of a carbohydrate-protein beverage on cycling endurance and muscle damage. *Medicine & Science in Sports & Exercise* 36 (7):1233-1238.

Shi, X., R.W. Summers, H.P. Schedl, S.W Flanagan., R. Chang and C.V. Gisolfi. 1995. Effects of carbohydrate type and concentration and solution osmolality on water absorption. *Medicine & Science in Sports & Exercise* 27:1607-1615.

Shirreffs, S.M., A.J. Taylor, J.B. Leiper and R.J. Maughan. 1996. Post-exercise rehydration in man—Effects of volume consumed and drink sodium content. *Medicine & Science in Sports & Exercise* 28 (10):1260-1271.

Vist, G.E., and R.J. Maughan. 1995. The effect of osmolality and carbohydrate content on the rate of gastric emptying of liquids in man. *Journal of Physiology* 486: 523-531.

Walsh, R.M., T.D. Noakes, J.A Hawley and S.C. Dennis. 1994. Impaired high-intensity cycling performance time at low levels of dehydration. *International Journal of Sports Medicine* 15:392-398.

Wilk, B., S. Kriemler, H. Keller and O. Bar-Or. 1998. Consistency in preventing voluntary dehydration in boys who drink a flavoured carbohydrate-NaCl beverage during exercise in the heat. *International Journal of Sport Nutrition* 8:1-9.

chapter six

Sherwood, L. 2001. *Human physiology.* 4th ed. Pacific Grove, CA: Brooks/Cole.

Whitney, E.R., and S. R. Rolfes. 2005. *Understanding nutrition.* 10th ed. Belmont, CA: Wadsworth.

chapter seven

Burke, L., and V. Deakin, eds. 2000. *Clinical sports nutrition.* 2nd ed. New York: McGraw-Hill.

Burke, L.M., G.R. Collier and S.K. Beasley. 1995. Effect of co-ingestion of fat and protein with CHO feedings on muscle glycogen storage. *Journal of Applied Physiology* 78:2187-2192.

Hawley, J.A., and L.M. Burke. 1997. Effect of meal frequency and timing on physical performance. *British Journal of Nutrition* 77 (Suppl):S91-S103.

Fallon, K.E., E. Broad, M.W. Thompson and P.A. Reull. 1998. Nutritional and fluid intake in a 100 km ultramarathon. *International Journal of Sport Nutrition* 8:24-35.

Ivy, J.L., H.W. Goforth, B.M. Damon, T.R. McCauley, E.C. Parsons and T.B. Price. 2002. Early postexercise muscle glycogen recovery is enhanced with a carbohydrate-protein supplement. *Journal of Applied Physiology* 93: 1337-1344.

Kang, J., R.J Robertson, B.G. Denys, S.G. DaSilva, P. Visich, R.R. Suminski., A.C. Utter, F.L. Goss and K.F. Metz. 1995. Effect of carbohydrate ingestion subsequent to carbohydrate supercompensation on endurance performance. *International Journal of Sport Nutrition* 5:329-343.

Lucia, A., C. Earnest and C. Arribas. 2003. The Tour de France: A physiological review. *Scandinavian Journal of Medicine and Science in Sports* 13:275-283.

MacDougall, J.D., G.R. Ward, D.G. Sale and J.R. Sutton. 1977. Muscle glycogen repletion after high intensity intermittent exercise. *Journal of Applied Physiology* 42 (2):129-132.

Saris, W.H. 1990. The Tour de France: Food intake and energy expenditure during extreme sustained exercise. *Cycling Science* 2 (4):17-21.

Stroud, M.A., P. Ritz, W.A. Coward, M.B. Sawyer, D. Constantin-Teodosiu, P.L. Greenhaff and I.A. Macdonald. 1997. Energy expenditure using isotope-labelled water (^{2}H$_2$ ^{18}O), exercise performance, skeletal muscle enzyme activities and plasma biochemical parameters in humans during 95 days of endurance exercise with inadequate energy intake. *European Journal of Applied Physiology* 76:243-252.

Ventura, J.L., A. Estruch, G. Rodas, and R. Segura. 1994. Effect of prior ingestion of glucose or fructose on the performance of exercise of intermediate duration. *European Journal of Applied Physiology* 68:345-349.

Zawadski, K.M., B.B. Yaspelkis and J.L. Ivy. 1992. Carbohydrate-protein complex increases the rate of muscle glycogen storage after exercise. *Journal of Applied Physiology* 72 (5):1854-1859.

chapter eight

Antonio, J., and J.R. Stout. 2002. *Supplements for endurance athletes.* Champaign, IL: Human Kinetics.

Antonio, J., and J.R. Stout. 2002. *Supplements for strength-power athletes.* Champaign, IL: Human Kinetics.

Armstrong, L.E. 2002. Caffeine, body fluid-electrolyte balance, and exercise performance. *International Journal of Sport Nutrition and Exercise Metabolism* 12:189-206.

Australian Institute of Sport. 2005. AIS Sports Supplement Program 2005. www.ais.org.au/nutrition/Supplements.asp.

Bahrke, M.S., and W.P. Morgan. 2002. Evaluation of the ergogenic properties of ginseng. *Sports Medicine* 29: 113-133.

Braun, B., P.M. Clarkson, P.S. Freedson and R.L. Kohl. 1991. Effects of co-enzyme Q10 supplementation on exercise performance, $\dot{V}O_2$max and lipid peroxidation in trained cyclists. *International Journal of Sport Nutrition* 1:353-365.

Brouns, F., and G.J. van der Vusse. 1998. Utilisation of lipids during exercise in human subjects: Metabolic and dietary constraints. *British Journal of Nutrition* 79: 117-128.

Burke, L. 1995. *The complete guide to food for sports performance.* London: Allen and Unwin.

Burke, L., and V. Deakin, eds. 2000. *Clinical sports nutrition.* 2nd ed. New York: McGraw-Hill.

Candow, D.G., P.D. Chilibeck, D.G. Burke, K.S. Davison and T. Smith-Palmer. 2001. Effect of glutamine supplementation combined with resistance training in young adults. *European Journal of Applied Physiology* 86:142-149.

Clancy, S.P., P.M. Clarkson, M.E. De Cheke, K. Nosaka, P.S. Freedson, J.J. Cunningham and B. Valentine. 1994. Effects of chromium picolinate supplementation on body composition, strength, and urinary chromium loss in football players. *International Journal of Sport Nutrition* 4:142-153.

Clarkson, P.M. 1996. Nutrition for improved sports performance. *Sports Medicine* 21:393-401.

Clarkson, P.M. 1997. Effects of exercise on chromium levels. *Sports Medicine* 23:341-349.

Dekkers J.C., L.J.P. van Doornen and C.G. Kemper. 1996. The role of antioxidant vitamins and enzymes in the prevention of exercise-induced muscle damage. *Sports Medicine* 21:213-238.

Engels, H.J. and J.C. Wirth. 1997. No ergogenic effects of ginseng (Panax ginseng) during graded maximal aerobic exercise. *Journal of the American Dietetic Association* 97:1110-1115.

Fiala, K.A., D.J. Casa and M.W. Roti. 2004. Rehydration with a caffeinated beverage during the non-exercise periods of 3 consecutive days of 2-a-day practices. *International Journal of Sport Nutrition and Exercise Metabolism* 14:419-429.

Fogelholm, G.M., H.K. Näveri, K.T.K. Kiilavuori and M.H.A. Härkönen. 1993. Low-dose amino acid supplementation: No effects on serum human growth hormone and insulin in male weightlifters. *International Journal of Sport Nutrition* 3:290-297.

Fricker, P.A., S.K. Beasley and I.W. Copeland. 1988. Physiological growth hormone responses of throwers to amino acids, eating and exercise. *Australian Journal of Science and Medicine in Sport* (March):21-23.

Greenhaff, P.L. 1995. Creatine and its application as an ergogenic aid. *International Journal of Sport Nutrition* 5: S100-S110.

Horswill, C.A. 1995. Effects of bicarbonate, citrate, and phosphate loading on performance. *International Journal of Sport Nutrition* 5:S111-S119.

Kanter, M. 1998. Free radicals, exercise and antioxidant supplementation. *Proceedings of the Nutrition Society* 57:9-13.

Kanter, M.M., and M.H. Williams. 1995. Antioxidants, carnitine, and choline as putative ergogenic aids. *International Journal of Sport Nutrition* 5 (Suppl):S120-S131.

Lambert, M.I., J. Hefer, R.P. Millar and P.W. Macfarlane. 1993. Failure of commercial oral amino acid supplements to increase serum growth hormone concentrations in male body builders. *International Journal of Sport Nutrition* 3:298-305.

Maughan, R. 2003, October. Dietary supplement use in sports. Re-energise Conference, Dudley, England.

Moffat, R.J., and S.A. Chelland. 2004. Carnitine. In *Nutritional ergogenic aids,* edited by I. Wolinsky and J.A. Driskell. Boca Raton, FL: CRC Press, pp. 61-79.

Nissen, S.L. 2004. Beta-hydroxy-beta-methylbutyrate. In *Nutritional ergogenic aids,* edited by I. Wolinsky and J.A. Driskell. Boca Raton, FL: CRC Press.

Powers, S.K., and K. Hamilton 1999. Antioxidants and exercise. *Clinics in Sports Medicine* 18:525-536.

Sport Dietary Supplement Update. 2005. Human Kinetics. www.humankinetics.com/sdsu/content/toc.cfm.

U.S. Food and Drug Administration Center for Food Safety and Applied Nutrition. March 2005. Consumer education and general information on dietary supplements. www.cfsan.fda.gov/~dms/ds-info.html.

Wemple, R.D, D.R. Lamb and K.H. McKeever. 1997. Caffeine vs caffeine-free sports drinks: Effects on urine production at rest and during prolonged exercise. *International Journal of Sports Medicine* 18:40-46.

Weston, S.B., S. Zhou, R.P. Weatherby and S.J. Robson. 1997. Does exogenous coenzyme Q10 affect aerobic capacity in endurance athletes? *International Journal of Sport Nutrition* 7:197-206.

Williams, M.H. 1998. *The ergogenics edge.* Champaign, IL: Human Kinetics.

Wolinsky, I., and J.A. Driskell. 2004. *Nutritional ergogenic aids.* Boca Raton, FL: CRC Press.

World Anti-Doping Agency. 2004. Dietary supplements Q&As. www.wada-ama.org/en/dynamic.ch2?pageCategory_id=99.

chapter ten

Australian Institute of Sport. 2004. AIS Sports Nutrition - Travel www.ais.org.au/nutrition/Travel.asp.

Burke, L. 1990. The travelling athlete. *Australian Fitness and Training* 5 (4):62-65.

Hill, D.W., C.M. Hill, K.L. Fields and J.C. Smith. 1993. Effects of jet lag on factors related to sport performance. *Canadian Journal of Applied Physiology* 18 (1):91-103.

Manfredini, R., F. Manfredini, C. Fersini and F. Conconi. 1998. Circadium rhythms, athletic performance, and jet lag. *British Journal Sports Medicine* 32:101-106.

Sports Dietitians Australia. 2000. Nutrition and the traveling athlete. Fact sheet #8. Melbourne: Sports Dietitians Australia. www.sportsdietitians.com.au/www/html/1935-nutrition-and-the-travelling-athlete.asp

Waterhouse, J., B. Edwards, A. Nevill, S. Carvalho, G. Atkinson, P. Buckley, T. Reilly, R. Godfrey and Ramsay, R. 2002. Identifying some determinants of 'jet lag' and its symptoms: A study of athletes and other travellers. *British Journal Sports Medicine* 36:54-60.

Youngstedt, S.D. and P.J. O'Connor. 1999. The influence of air travel on athletic performance. *Sports Medicine* 28:197-207.

chapter eleven

Antonio, J., and J.R. Stout. 2002. *Supplements for strength-power athletes.* Champaign, IL: Human Kinetics.

Balon, T.W., J.F. Horowitz and K.M. Fitzsimmons. 1992. Effects of carbohydrate loading and weight lifting on muscle girth. *International Journal of Sport Nutrition* 2: 328-334.

Børsheim, E., A. Aarsland and R.R. Wolfe. 2004. Effect of an amino acid, protein, and carbohydrate mixture on net muscle protein balance after resistance exercise. *International Journal of Sport Nutrition and Exercise Metabolism* 14:255-271.

Fussell, S. 1991. *Muscle.* London: Cardinal.

Kreider, R.B. 1999. Dietary supplements and the promotion of muscle growth with resistance exercise. *Sports Medicine* 27:97-110.

Lambert, C.P., L.L. Frank and W.J. Evans. 2004. Macronutrient considerations for the sport of bodybuilding. *Sports Medicine* 34:317-327.

Walberg-Rankin, J. 1995. A review of nutritional practices and needs of bodybuilders. *Journal of Strength and Conditioning Research* 9 (2):116-124.

Wolinsky, I., and J.A. Driskell. 2004. *Nutritional ergogenic aids.* Boca Raton, FL: CRC Press.

chapter twelve

Astrup, A., M.T. Larsen and A. Harper. 2004. Atkins and other low-carbohydrate diets: Hoax or an effective tool for weight loss? *Lancet* 364:897-899.

Beals, K.A., and M.M. Manore. 1994. The prevalence and consequences of subclinical eating disorders in female athletes. *International Journal of Sport Nutrition* 4:175-195.

Bravata, D.M., L. Sanders, J. Huang, H.M. Krumholz, I. Olkin, C.D. Gardner and D.M. Bravata. 2003. Efficacy and safety of low-carbohydrate diets. *Journal of the American Medical Association* 289:1837-1850.

Bray, G.A., and B.M. Popkin. 1998. Dietary fat intake does effect obesity! *American Journal of Clinical Nutrition* 68: 1157-1173.

Food and Agriculture Organisation of the United Nations. 1998. Report of a Joint FAO/WHO Expert Consultation. Carbohydrates in human nutrition. FAO Food and Nutrition Paper. Rome: Food and Agriculture Organisation.

Gades, D.M. and J.S. Stern. 2003. Chitosan supplementation and fecal fat excretion in men. *Obesity Research* 11: 683-688.

Fogelholm, M. 1994. Effects of bodyweight reduction on sports performance. *Sports Medicine* 18 (4):248-267.

Holt, S.H.A., J.C. Brand-Miller, P. Petocz and E. Farmaka-lidis. 1995. A satiety index of common foods. *European Journal of Clinical Nutrition* 49:675-690.

Jeukendrup, A., and M. Gleeson. 2004. *Sport nutrition.* Champaign, IL: Human Kinetics.

Lukin, Dean. *The Dean Lukin Diet.* 1993. Sydney: Margaret Gee Publishing.

Manore, M., and J. Thompson. 2000. *Sport nutrition for health and performance.* Champaign, IL: Human Kinetics.

Movahedi, A. 1999. Simple formula for calculating basal energy expenditure. *Nutrition Research* 19:989-995.

Ni Mhurchu, C., S.D. Poppitt, A.-T. McGill, F.E. Leahy, D.A. Bennett, B.B. Lin, D. Ormrod, I. Ward, C. Strik and A. Rodgers. 2004. The effect of the dietary supplement, Chitosan, on body weight: A randomized controlled trial in 250 overweight and obese adults. *International Journal of Obesity* 28:1149-1156.

Rolls, B.J., and E.A. Bell. 1999. Intake of fat and carbohy-drate: Role of energy density. *European Journal of Clinical Nutrition* 53:S166-S173.

Rosenbaum, M., V. Prieto, J. Hellmer, M. Boschmann, J. Krueger, R. Leibel and A. Ship. 1998. An exploratory investigation of the morphology and biochemistry of cellulite. *Plastic and Reconstructive Surgery* 101:1934-1939.

Rossi, A.B.R., and A.L. Vergnanini. 2000. Cellulite: A review. *Journal of the European Academy of Dermatology and Venerology* 14:251-262.

Sherwood, L. 2001. *Human physiology.* 4th ed. Pacific Grove, CA: Brooks/Cole.

Sports Dietitians Australia. September 2001. Fact sheet #14: Eating disorders in athletes. Melbourne: Sports Dietitians Australia.

Sundgot-Borgen, J. 1994. Eating disorders in female ath-letes. *Sports Medicine* 17 (3):176-188.

Taber's Cyclopedic Medical Dictionary. 2001. 19th ed. Phila-delphia: F.A. Davis Company.

US Department of Health and Human Services and the US Department of Agriculture. Dietary guide-lines for Americans. 2005. www.healthierus.gov/dietaryguidelines.

Wing, R.R., and J.O. Hill. 2001. Successful weight loss maintenance. *Annual Reviews of Nutrition* 21:323-341.

Wichman, S., and D.R. Martin. 1993. Eating disorders in athletes. *Physician and Sportsmedicine* 21 (5):126-135.

resources

Recommended Reading

Antonio, J., and J.R. Stout. 2002. *Supplements for endurance athletes*. Champaign IL: Human Kinetics.

Antonio, J., and J.R. Stout. 2002. *Supplements for strength-power athletes*. Champaign, IL: Human Kinetics.

Brand-Miller, J., K. Foster-Powell and S. Colaguiri. 2002. *The new glucose revolution*. Sydney: Hodder.

Burke, L. 1995. *The complete guide to food for sports performance*. London: Allen and Unwin.

Burke, L., and V. Deakin, eds. 2000. *Clinical sports nutrition*. New York: McGraw-Hill.

Hawley, J., and L. Burke. 1998. *Peak performance*. London: Allen and Unwin.

Jeukendrup, A., and M. Gleeson. 2004. *Sport nutrition*. Champaign, IL: Human Kinetics.

Manore, M., and J. Thompson. 2000. *Sport nutrition for health and performance*. Champaign, IL: Human Kinetics.

Rolls, B., and R.A. Barnett. 2000. *Volumetrics weight control plan*. New York: Quill.

Saxelby, C. 2002. *Nutrition for life*. 4th ed. South Yarra, Australia: Hardie Grant Books.

Stear, S. 2004. *Fuelling fitness for sports performance*. London: The Sugar Bureau (UK).

For books on all aspects of sports science, including sports nutrition, contact Human Kinetics in your country for a catalogue or go to www.HumanKinetics.com.

Sports Nutrition and General Nutrition Web Sites

American Dietetic Association

www.eatright.org
Go to the 'Food and Nutrition Information' section for good-quality resources.

Australian Institute of Sport Department of Sports Nutrition

www.ais.org.au/nutrition/index.asp
This site has everything—stuff on supplements, recipes, resources and, of course, sports nutrition.

British Dietetic Association

www.bda.uk.com
The home of dietitians in the UK. Check out their 'Latest Food Facts' section.

Dietitians Association of Australia

www.daa.asn.au
This site has lots of useful general nutrition information for the public.

Dietitians in Sport and Exercise Nutrition (UK)

www.disen.org
This site has the basics of sports nutrition and tips on popular sports.

Freelance Dietitians Group of the British Dietetic Association

www.dietitiansunlimited.co.uk
Use this site to find a sports dietitian in the UK.

Gatorade Sports Science Institute

www.gssiweb.com
A good-quality site for sports nutrition issues with a bent toward sports drinks.

Glenn Cardwell

www.glenncardwell.com
On this site you will find a range of e-books, nutrition articles, free newsletter, books and products . . . and all you wanted to know about chocolate! Subscribe to the free newsletter.

Lucozade Sports Science

www.lucozadesport.com
This site has lots of information on sports drinks and sports nutrition.

Nutrition Australia

www.nutritionaustralia.org
Information produced by nutrition professionals. Subscribe to their free online newsletter and check their FAQs on nutrition.

Sport Dietetics—United States

www.scandpg.org

This is the Web site of sports dietitians in the United States. It provides nutrition advice and manuals.

Sports Dietitians Australia

www.sportsdietitians.com.au
Click on 'Fact Sheets' for free sports nutrition pdf files. Also has information on nutrition for different sports. Produced for the general public by sports dietitians.

index

Note: The italicized f and t following page numbers refer to figures and tables, respectively.

about the author

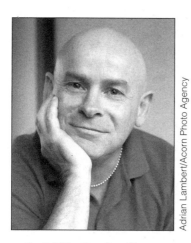

Adrian Lambert/Acorn Photo Agency

Glenn Cardwell is a qualified sports dietitian and an accredited practising dietitian with more than 25 years of experience. He has advised athletes from junior ranks through elite levels, and he has run courses for fitness leaders and personal trainers since 1986. One of the first sports dietitians in Australia, he lectures in sports nutrition at Edith Cowan University.

Cardwell helped to establish Sports Dietitians Australia, a professional body of qualified sports dietitians, and serves as their newsletter editor. He was the sports nutrition adviser to the West Coast Eagles (Australian Football League) for 14 seasons. Now he is with Western Force (Super 14 Rugby League). He has written many articles on sports nutrition for magazines and professional newsletters.

In 2002, Cardwell was privileged to accompany Australian fast bowler Brett Lee to Chicago to study his sweat composition and losses. In 2003, Cardwell was made a life member of Nutrition Australia for services to nutrition education. He was judged Professional Speaker of the Year by the National Speakers Association of Australia (WA Chapter).

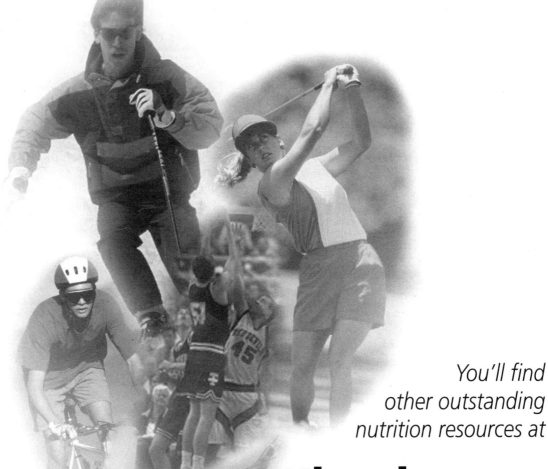